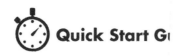 **Quick Start G**

MW00450889

What Can I Eat?
ON A
GLUTEN-FREE
DIET

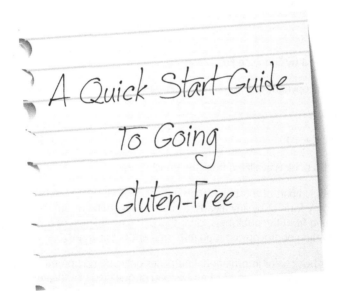

A Quick Start Guide
To Going
Gluten-Free

Lose Weight, Feel Great
and Increase Your Energy!

PLUS over 100 Delicious Gluten-Free Recipes

First published in 2014 by Erin Rose Publishing

Text and illustration copyright © 2014 Erin Rose Publishing

Design: Julie Anson

ISBN: 978-0-9928232-5-2

A CIP record for this book is available from the British Library.

DISCLAIMER: This book is for informational purposes only and not intended as a substitute for the medical advice, diagnosis or treatment of a physician or qualified healthcare provider. The reader should consult a physician before undertaking a new health care regimen and in all matters relating to his/her health, and particularly with respect to any symptoms that may require diagnosis or medical attention.

While every care has been taken in compiling the recipes for this book we cannot accept responsibility for any problems which arise as a result of preparing one of the recipes. The author and publisher disclaim responsibility for any adverse effects that may arise from the use or application of the recipes in this book. Some of the recipes in this book include nuts and eggs. If you have an egg or nut allergy it's important to avoid these. It is recommended that children, pregnant women, the elderly or anyone who has an immune system disorder avoid eating raw eggs.

CONTENTS

Recipes

INTRODUCTION

Have you been finding you wake in the morning with a flat tummy but by the afternoon your trousers are tight and your stomach feels twice the size? Or perhaps your belly bloat just won't go away no matter what you do? It's time to look into the possibility that gluten, the sticky protein in wheat, could be to blame. For some people, gluten can play havoc with their digestion and cause a range of problems, as well as the more obvious bloating. Often the only real way to tell if you are intolerant to gluten is to eliminate it from your diet and look at the results.

In this **Quick Start Guide** we take a comprehensive approach and give you the information you need to easily remove gluten from your diet and improve your digestion, wellbeing and vitality. A gluten-free diet can make a vast different to your weight, your health and it also opens you up to a whole range of exciting ways of eating which you may not have experienced before. To help you to make these changes, we have included plenty of easy and delicious recipes to make it simple to incorporate these into your everyday life. A gluten-free diet doesn't have to feel restrictive. You can maintain variety, enjoy great flavours and eat healthy nutritious food which is easy to prepare.

The thought of eliminating common staples from your diet may be really daunting, and it can deter people from taking the first step because they don't know what else to eat. But our mission is to make it easy for you and to show you how to attain your goal without feeling deprived – once you feel the difference then you can decide whether to sustain your gluten-free diet.

Should I Go Gluten-Free?

If you are looking into the benefits of a gluten-free diet the chances are you already suspect that gluten is causing you a problem. The effects of gluten can range from mild to severe; from gluten intolerance to coeliac disease which has considerable health implications. We have included a symptom checker, to help you ascertain if gluten is causing you a problem. It isn't intended to replace medical diagnosis, but it will provide you with sufficient insight into the ways gluten could be affecting you. Most importantly, you'll learn what you can do about it!

What Is Gluten?

So we know that gluten is a protein found in wheat but it's also found in rye, barley and oats too. Apart from obvious wheat and flour based foods like bread, cakes, biscuits, cookies, crackers and breakfast cereals, gluten is also found in foods derived from glutinous grains such as thickeners, sauces and malt vinegar.

The word gluten is a Latin word meaning 'glue' which is also an apt description of what happens when you combine flour and water together. Mixing together 1 part flour and 2 parts water was an old fashioned way to make glue. So with that in mind we can get an insight into what is happening inside our intestines when we eat products made with glutinous flour. For many of us a 'normal' diet consists of toast for breakfast, a sandwich for lunch an evening meal possibly consisting of pasta, noodles or pizza, so gluten can easily be consumed 3 times a day, if not more!

Coeliacs suffer an auto immune response to gluten, and know all too well the harmful effect is has on them, resulting in malabsorption, malnutrition and anaemia if they continue to eat it.

Approximately 1% of the population is diagnosed with coeliac disease, a chronic auto immune disorder where the body attacks itself, causing harm to the gut lining when the invading gluten enters it. If you have coeliac disease it is more likely that you could also develop lactose intolerance due to the lack of enzymes affecting your ability to digest dairy produce.

However, let's remember the negative effects of gluten are not limited to those with diagnosed coeliac disease. In fact gluten 'sensitivity' is much more common. It's thought that as many as 6-7% of people are sensitive to the effects of gluten, resulting in problems with their digestion, such as diarrhoea, bloating, wind and abdominal pain. Wheat is considered to be one of the top food allergens. That isn't good news if it's a huge part of your daily diet which, for many of us, it is.

While there is a medical test for coeliac disease, there is no accurate test for gluten intolerance. Unlike coeliac disease, which is caused by an auto immune response, gluten sensitivity is caused by an allergy or intolerance. However the symptoms of the 2 disorders are very similar. The important difference between them is that in a non-coeliac person with gluten sensitivity, there doesn't appear to be damage to the gut lining. However in coeliac disease, the gut wall deteriorates due to the immune response and destroys its ability to absorb nutrients in the small intestine. Furthermore gluten intolerance and coeliac disease are both on the rise, yet there is no definitive reason for this. It's thought that the increased consumption of wheat as an ingredient in processed foods may be contributing, or the fact that wheat has been hybridized to contain more gluten than it used to. On the plus side there is a ray of sunshine – gluten has NO nutritional benefit! So once it's removed from your diet, the only way is up!

Symptom Checker

- Diarrhoea.

- Bloating.

- Gas.

- Constipation.

- Stomach pain.

- Joint pain.

- Skin rashes.

- Migraines.

- Foggy thinking.

- Unexplained infertility.

- Urticaria (hives).

- Recurring nasal congestion.

- Failure to thrive in children.

- Low iron levels.

If you suffer from any of the above, discuss it with your doctor who may perform a coeliac test. Even if it comes back negative, it's worth removing gluten from your diet and monitoring any changes to your symptoms.

IMPORTANT RED FLAGS!

It's vitally important to see your doctor if you have any of the following:

- Blood in your stools
- Unexplained weight loss
- Any changes to your normal bowel habit which lasts longer than 4 weeks.

What Can I Do About It?

Cut out gluten. But if only it were that simple, right? The substance is in so many of our food products, not just bread, cakes and pasta. Gluten is also a sneaky addition to sausages, some cured meats, ready meals and pre-made sauces. If you are gluten sensitive, just how much of an impact gluten is having on you will really only be known when you cut it out of your diet. To do this you'll need to be aware of product labelling and the unexpected ingredients in some of your favourite foods and condiments, like vinegar and soy sauce. For coeliacs who are severely affected, cross-contamination is a real concern because even a minute amount can cause a problem.

For that reason it's worth taking extra care and keeping some kitchen equipment separate and use a different toaster for gluten-free bread. It's accepted worldwide that products with the Crossed Grain symbol signify that a product is gluten-free and is safe for coeliacs to eat. If you have been diagnosed with coeliac disease, go gluten-free as soon as you are diagnosed. Please note that going gluten-free before a coeliac test can result in a false negative. If however you suspect that you are gluten intolerant, try going gluten-free for one month and monitor the changes. You may notice greater mental clarity and a reduction in your waistline.

Seriously, you have nothing to lose and everything to gain. By cutting out gluten for 1 month it will give you a chance to gauge how much you are being affected. If at the end of the month you are still doubtful, re-introduce gluten into your diet and see what happens. If your symptoms return then stick with being gluten-free. It may seem awkward when you first try removing gluten but once you are into the swing of it and know what you can eat it will be a lot easier.

Keeping a food diary and a record of how you feel in terms of, bloating, gas, bowel habits etc; will give you a really good indicator of what is affecting you. Remember to keep that diary going if you do decide to re-introduce gluten and write down what happens. It really is up to you how much you stick to it. But if returning to your old patterns causes an avalanche of symptoms, get back into your gluten-free eating pattern. Once you know that you are allowing the symptoms to affect you it'll give you impetus to keep going. It'll justify the short term challenges and you'll have the answers you need.

Oats – Gluten-Free Or Not Gluten-Free

Strictly speaking oats don't contain gluten, however they are usually processed in a factory with glutinous grains, therefore there is a strong chance they are cross-contaminated and can't be classified gluten-free. However oats do contain avenin, a substance similar to gluten which is also a protein. A small number of people also have a problem with avenin.

This is where the 1 month test really comes into play. After 1 month on a gluten-free detox, sample oats and see how you feel. If you know they aren't good for you based on how they then make you feel, give them a wide berth. It is possible to get certified gluten-free oats, however be aware that a small minority of people can still be intolerant to them.

What Can I Eat?

Don't eat these:

- Wheat
- Durum wheat
- Rye
- Barley
- Semolina
- Bulgur wheat
- Farina
- Graham flour
- Kamut
- Triticale (a cross between rye and wheat)
- Spelt
- Oats, unless certified gluten-free

AVOID these unless the label states 'gluten free'

- Flour: bread, batter coatings, breaded coatings, bagels, tortillas, pizza, cookies, wraps, pitta bread, muesli, granola, biscuits, pancakes and crackers
- Pasta
- Bread
- Bran
- Couscous
- Noodles

- Semolina

- Burgers, sausages, marinated meats and luncheon meat

- Certain salad dressings and spice blends

- Readymade and canned soups

- Flavoured roasted nuts

- Battered or breaded fish, onion rings, coated chicken and processed meats which contain rusk

- Pickles & chutneys

- Stock (broth) cubes, salad dressings

- Modified starch - check for the source of the starch or avoid it

- Certain medications and vitamin supplements which are bound with gluten

AVOID any products derived from gluten grains:

- Malt vinegar

- Barley malt

- Malt flavourings

- Soy sauce, marinades, gravy mixes, stock (broth) and readymade sauces

- Beer, ale & lager

What Can I Eat?

You can eat these:

- Gluten free flours ie: rice, corn, chickpea (garbanzo bean), potato, soya, coconut, almond flour and all nut flours.

- Corn and corn meal

- Polenta

- Buckwheat

- Flaxseed

- Arrowroot

- Rice noodles

- Sorghum

- Garfava

- Quinoa

- Millet

- Amaranth

- Kasha

- Teff flour

- Potato starch

- Arrowroot starch

- Cornflour or Cornstarch

- Polenta

- Potatoes

- Corn

- Wheatgrass - it really is gluten-free!

- Vegetables

- Fruit

- Pulses, seeds and nuts

- Fresh unprocessed meat, poultry and seafood

- Eggs

- Dairy products, yogurt, cheese, milk

- Oils and butter

- Honey, sugar and syrup

- Pepper, salt, fresh herbs & spices

- Wine & champagne

- Tea & Coffee - beware of flavoured drinks with barley malt though

- Distilled red and white vinegar (not malt vinegar!)

Note: Wheat-free does not mean gluten-free because rye, barley and oats may still be present. Something is considered gluten-free if it has less than 20 parts per million (ppm) of gluten. The Crossed Grain symbol is internationally recognised by consumers as being gluten-free. It is a registered trademark and can only be used under licence by food and drink companies who meet the criteria.

Shopping And Eating Out

Once you get to know what you are shopping for it won't present too much of a challenge but getting to that point can be a steep learning curve. To make life easier there are now apps available which provide a directory of branded food and drink, to tell you if something is suitable for a gluten-free diet or not. What's more is these apps can guide you to the restaurants which cater for gluten-free diets and you can check out their menus too.

So if you are shopping you needn't be stumped by the labelling, you can check the app before buying. Reading the label is so important and if you are still in doubt you can call the manufacturer for clarification.

Tips To Make It Easy

- Have a separate toaster, utensils and chopping board for gluten-free bread

- Keep gluten-free products in their own storage containers

- Be scrupulous about utensils or even better keep separate coloured utensils to prevent mishaps with contamination

- Check your medication for gluten – ask your pharmacist if you're not sure

- Be aware that some vitamin and mineral supplements can contain gluten

- Find a tasty gluten-free bouillon or stock (broth) cubes

- Be careful of cooked ham - not just the crumbed variety. During slicing hams can become cross-contaminated

- Be vigilant when buying low-fat foods, especially yogurt which can be thickened with a gluten-containing starch

- Prepare some tasty meals and treats for the fridge or freezer. Have something gluten-free close by so that you aren't tempted

- If you are having cravings because one of your favourite things contains gluten, try finding a gluten-free alternative or try snacking on something else to break the habit

- Nuts, seeds and olives are quick and easy snacks which are high in protein – great for breaking a carb habit too!

- Rice cakes are a great staple and they go with just about anything

The Cheat Sheet

Sometimes you need to be creative when you're going gluten-free and with this in mind we have provided a cheat sheet to give you tasty alternatives.

The Substitutes

Courgette (Zucchini) Ribbons For Pasta

Using a vegetable peeler, or spiralizer gadget, cut strips off the courgette and fry them until soft and serve instead of a bed of pasta. You can also try it with carrots or aubergines (eggplants) for a 'spaghetti' twist. Alternatively serve your Bolognese onto a plateful of fresh, green, leafy vegetables like baby spinach.

Gluten-Free Oats For Breadcrumbs

Make a breadcrumb substitute by combining some gluten-free rolled oats with some dried herbs and use it to dip your meat into before cooking.

Ground almonds, also known as almond flour or almond meal are a great alternative to breadcrumbs. You can coat fish or chicken in it for a delicious variation. Alternatively flaxseeds (linseeds) whizzed in a blender with some dried herbs make a healthy and tasty alternative to breadcrumbs.

Chopped Nuts For Croutons

Who doesn't like soup with crispy croutons? But you needn't feel like you're missing out. Chop some walnuts, pecans, brazil nuts or almonds and scatter on top of your favourite soup. For added flavour you can toast them first and add a sprinkling of cinnamon, chilli powder or salt.

Rice Noodles For Wheat Noodles

Instead of traditional wheat and egg noodles, substitute with rice noodles which are readily available in most supermarkets. Remember to double check that they are gluten-free.

Lettuce Leaves For Tortilla Wraps

Use romaine or iceberg lettuce leaves instead of a bread wrap. Simply scoop your chilli or similar meat dish into the lettuce leaf, add guacamole, cheese and you have a taco which is not only gluten-free but also low carb.

You could also try a corn tortilla but check that it really is gluten-free.

Popcorn For Potato Crisps/Potato Chips

If your favourite potato crisps/chips contain wheat in the seasoning and you can't get the guarantee that plain crisps are gluten-free, try popcorn instead. Buy the corn ready to pop, cook it and then add your own seasoning – a little sea salt, chilli, cinnamon or even garlic salt gives it a lift.

Cauliflower For Couscous

Place some raw cauliflower into a blender and blitz it. You can eat it raw or lightly fry it with a little olive oil. Using vegetables to replace some of the carbohydrates in our meals is pretty exciting and just takes a little imagination.

Cornflour (Cornstarch) As A Thickener For Soups & Casseroles

Simply mix together equal quantities of cornflour and water in a cup then add to your recipe. Begin with 1-2 tablespoons of each and mix to a smooth paste before stirring into a soup or casserole.

Potatoes And Courgettes (Zucchini) For Soup Thickener

Potatoes and courgette (zucchini) also make great natural vegetable thickeners. Even if the recipe doesn't call for it, you can add a little of either vegetable which will likely go unnoticed, but it'll give it a creamy richness.

The True Test

A Month Of Gluten-Free Living

So the first step is to go gluten-free for one month. Once you have been gluten-free for a month you come to the next stage. However, this is entirely optional and provided you have stuck to being gluten-free for 30 days at least!

The most accurate way to see if cutting out gluten benefits you is to stop all consumption of it to allow your body to detox. You will be able to see for yourself if your bloating, bowel habits, weight, vitality, clarity and general health have improved, but perhaps you are still having doubts. Maybe you would have felt better anyhow? OK so the simple answer is to test yourself.

Add into your diet one item which contains gluten; a cracker or slice of bread - the simpler the better. If you think you have other intolerances make sure you have singled them out from your test food. Once you have eaten the test food, see if you notice any difference. It may be immediate or it may take 24/48 hours. Your food diary can really help you here. If you have felt better you may have forgotten about a symptom which has disappeared and it may flare up again with the test food, but you might not link it to the gluten. Please, this only applies if you are non-coeliac. Coeliacs should avoid gluten completely. It's not worth playing around and experiencing a relapse in symptoms if you KNOW you shouldn't have gluten.

So this step is optional, but it will provide you with the answer you've been looking for if you've suspected that you are gluten intolerant. It'll provide you with the information you need to decide if you wish to carry on being gluten-free and make it part of your normal healthy lifestyle. We wish you good luck, good health and we hope you enjoy the recipes!

All the recipes contained in this book are gluten-free and we have provided alternatives to using gluten-free flour too. Shop bought substitutes like stock cubes (broth), bread, biscuits, cookies and pasta are available but we wanted to give you a wide variety of options and make the recipes as healthy and delicious as possible.

When it comes to making stock (broth) there are options. There is a range of gluten-free bouillon and stock cubes on the market which are very handy to have in your cupboards. Some of the pre-made bouillon can have a high amount of salt or it may simply not be to your taste, so we have included two recipes for stock (broth); one is chicken and the other vegetable. You can make a large batch and freeze it into small portions and keep it until you are ready to use it. That way you know exactly what has gone into it and you can adjust it to your taste. So in our recipes use whichever you prefer – just keep it gluten-free.

In some of the soups there is an option to use just water in place of stock. This is because some of them are already so tasty and creamy that you may not need to add extra flavour or texture, so we've given you a choice.

We hope you really enjoy the recipes, have fun experimenting and finding your own favourites.

BREAKFAST

Spanish Tortilla

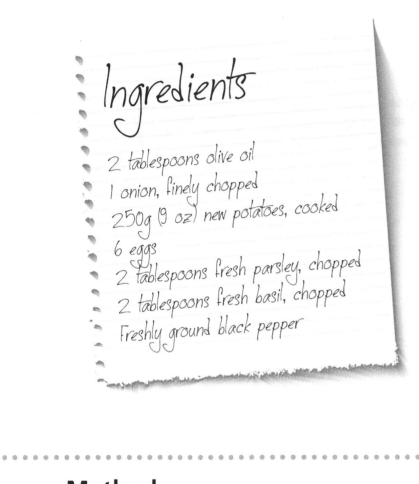

Ingredients

- 2 tablespoons olive oil
- 1 onion, finely chopped
- 250g (9 oz) new potatoes, cooked
- 6 eggs
- 2 tablespoons fresh parsley, chopped
- 2 tablespoons fresh basil, chopped
- Freshly ground black pepper

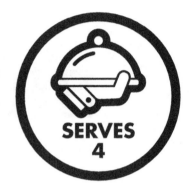

SERVES 4

Method

Heat the oil in a frying pan. Add the onion and cook until soft. Add the potatoes and warm through. In a separate bowl, whisk the eggs then add the parsley, basil and pepper. Pour the mixture into the pan on top of the onions and potatoes. Stir briefly then allow let it cook for around 3 minutes until it is set. When you are sure it is cooked through, place a plate on top of the pan and tip it out. Serve with salad. It can be served warm or cold and makes a great lunch box option.

Creamy Raspberry Oatmeal

Ingredients

2 tablespoons certified gluten-free oats

150g (5oz or 1 cup) raspberries, plus 3 or 4 for garnish

3 tablespoons natural yogurt (unflavoured)

SERVES
1

Method

Soak the oats in ½ cup boiling water for around 10 minutes. Place the oats in a blender, adding the raspberries and yogurt. Blend until smooth. Pour the raspberry mixture into a tall glass and top with a few raspberries. Serve and eat straight away.

Granola

Ingredients

150g (5oz or 1 cup) raw almonds, chopped
150g (5oz or 1 cup) raw walnuts, chopped
150g (5oz or 1 cup) raw pecans, chopped
75g (2 1/2 oz or 1/2 cup) desiccated (shredded) coconut
75g (2 1/2 oz or 1/2 cup) sunflower seeds
75g (2 1/2 oz or 1/2 cup) sultanas
75g (2 1/2 oz or 1/2 cup) ground flaxseed or flaxseed meal
1/2 teaspoon sea salt
120ml (4fl oz or 1/2 cup) coconut oil
4 tablespoons honey

Method

Grease and line a baking sheet with grease-proof paper. Melt the coconut oil and mix it with the honey. Add it to the nuts, coconut, seeds, and salt. Mix it together in a bowl and turn out onto the baking sheet. Scatter in an even layer. Bake at 150C/300F for 30-40 minutes. During baking stir the mixture twice to make sure it bakes evenly. Cook until lightly browned. Allow it to cool. Add in the sultanas and store in an airtight container. Serve the granola with natural yogurt, milk or it's equally delicious eaten on its own as a snack.

Apple Soufflé Omelette

SERVES 2

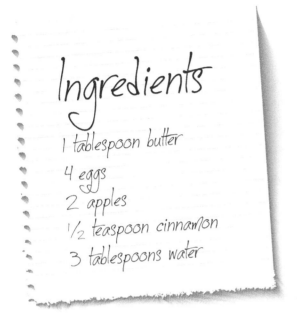

Ingredients

1 tablespoon butter

4 eggs

2 apples

1/2 teaspoon cinnamon

3 tablespoons water

Method

Peel, core and chop the apples. Place them in a saucepan with the water and cook for 5-10 minutes until they soften then mash with a fork. Once softly stewed add the cinnamon and stir. Set aside. Separate the egg yolks from the white and keep the yolks in a separate bowl while you whisk the egg whites into soft peaks. Then fold the yolks into the mixture.

Heat the butter in a small frying pan and add the whisked egg mixture. Cook the omelette until the eggs have set. It should be light and fluffy. Serve open on a plate, add the stewed apple and fold over. Eat straight away. As a variation you can try this recipe with raspberries or blueberries and a sprinkling of coconut.

Cheese & Ham Mini Omelettes

SERVES 4

Ingredients

4 large eggs
100g (3 ½ oz) Cheddar cheese, grated
50g (2oz or ¼ cup) ham, chopped
1 large tomato, chopped
Freshly ground black pepper

Method

Whisk the eggs then add the cheese, ham, tomato and black pepper. Lightly grease a muffin tin. Pour in the egg mixture. Bake on the top shelf of the oven at 180C/350F for around 20 minutes until the eggs are set. A huge variety of fillings can be used in this recipe; chicken & courgette, bacon & cheese, turkey & spinach, green pepper & chilli – the possibilities are endless.

Mexican Omelette

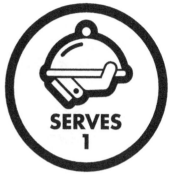

SERVES 1

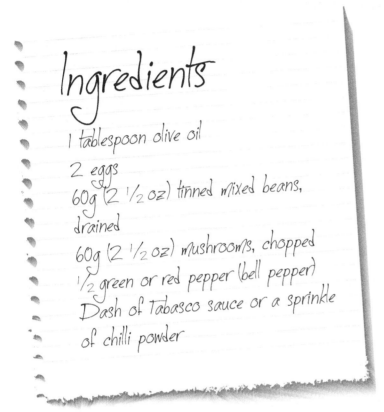

Ingredients

1 tablespoon olive oil

2 eggs

60g (2 ½ oz) tinned mixed beans, drained

60g (2 ½ oz) mushrooms, chopped

½ green or red pepper (bell pepper)

Dash of Tabasco sauce or a sprinkle of chilli powder

Method

Heat the olive oil in a pan. Add the mushrooms, peppers and beans. Cook for 3-4 minutes until the vegetables have softened. Remove them and set aside. Whisk the eggs in a bowl and pour them into the pan. Once the eggs begin to set, return the mushrooms, peppers and beans and spread them onto the eggs. Sprinkle with chilli or Tabasco sauce. Serve and eat straight away.

Spinach & Egg Breakfast Pots

SERVES 4

Ingredients

4 large eggs

60g (2 ½ oz) spinach

2 teaspoons olive oil

2 garlic clove, crushed

1 teaspoon paprika

1 tablespoon crème fraiche

Sea salt

Freshly ground black pepper

Method

Heat the olive oil in a pan. Add the garlic and paprika. When the garlic starts to soften, add the spinach. Cook for 2-3 minutes until the spinach is wilted. Divide the spinach and garlic between 4 ramekin dishes then break an egg into each one. Spoon some of the crème fraiche over each egg and sprinkle with paprika, salt and pepper. Place the ramekins in a preheated oven at 220C/425F for 15 minutes, until the eggs are set. Serve and enjoy.

Vegetable & Egg Rosti

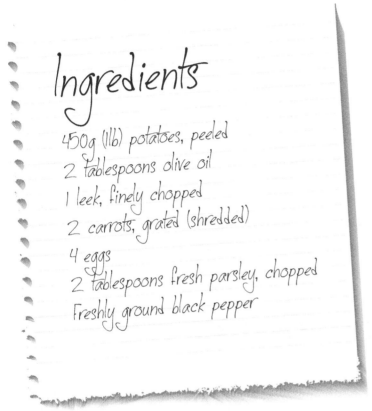

Ingredients

450g (1lb) potatoes, peeled
2 tablespoons olive oil
1 leek, finely chopped
2 carrots, grated (shredded)
4 eggs
2 tablespoons fresh parsley, chopped
Freshly ground black pepper

SERVES 4

Method

Grate (shred) the potatoes. Squeeze out the liquid using your hands and pat dry with a paper towel. Heat the olive oil in a frying pan. Add the leek and cook for 1 minute. Add the grated (shredded) carrots and potatoes, spreading them out in the pan. Cook for 10 minutes until crisp and golden. In the meantime, preheat the grill. Place the frying pan under the grill and cook until golden on top. Use the back of a spoon and make 4 egg-size indentations in the rosti. Crack an egg into each of them. Sprinkle with parsley and season with black pepper. Return the frying pan to the cooker and fry for 4-5 minutes until the eggs are cooked.

Spinach & Apple Smoothie

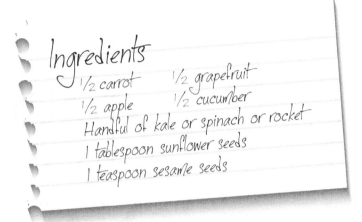

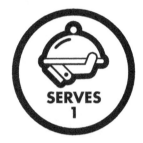

SERVES
1

Method

Place all of the ingredients into a high-powered blender, cover with water and blitz until smooth. If you're blender can't process seeds, they can be bought milled and added to the processed smoothie.

Banana & Avocado Smoothie

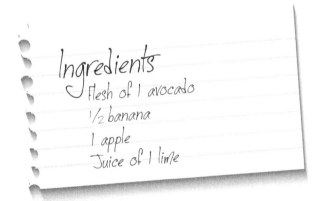

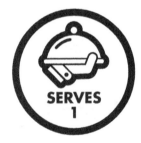

SERVES
1

Method

Put all the ingredients into a blender with just enough water to cover the ingredients. Blitz until smooth. It's frothy and delicious.

Apple & Ginger Smoothie

Ingredients

1 carrot
3 apples
1 cm (½ inch) chunk of root ginger

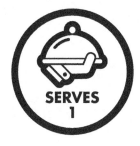

SERVES 1

Method

Place all the ingredients into a juice extractor and process or add the ingredients to a blender with enough water to cover.

Pina Colada Smoothie

Ingredients

½ small pineapple
240ml (8fl oz) coconut milk
Some crushed ice

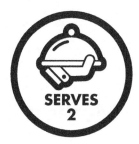

SERVES 2

Method

Put all the ingredients into a blender or food processor and blitz until smooth. Pour and enjoy.

Gluten-Free Pancakes

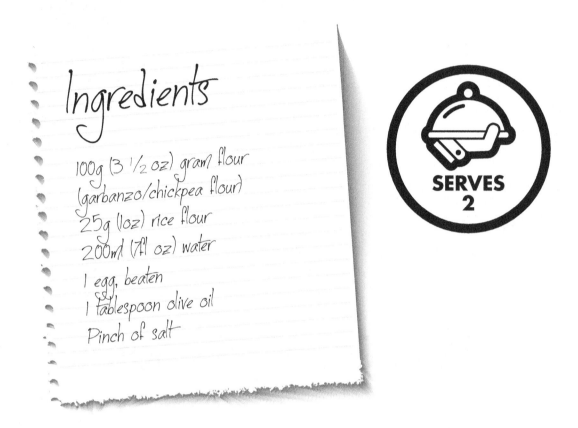

Ingredients

100g (3 ½ oz) gram flour
(garbanzo/chickpea flour)
25g (1oz) rice flour
200ml (7fl oz) water
1 egg, beaten
1 tablespoon olive oil
Pinch of salt

SERVES
2

Method

Place the gram flour and rice flour, salt, egg and water into a blender and process until smooth. Allow the mixture to stand for 10 minutes. Heat the olive oil in a frying pan. Add a little of the pancake mixture into the pan and cook for 2-3 minutes on each side. The mixture should make 4 large pancakes or 8 small ones.

Coconut & Almond Pancakes

SERVES 2

Ingredients

2 eggs
50g (2oz or ½ cup) almond flour
50g (2oz or ½ cup) rice flour
1 tablespoon desiccated (shredded) coconut
1 teaspoon coconut oil
1 teaspoon baking powder

Method

Whisk the eggs and set aside. Add the dry ingredients to a large bowl. Combine the whisked eggs into the dry ingredients, stirring until the batter becomes smooth. Heat a teaspoon of coconut oil in a frying pan. Spoon some of the mixture into the pan. Smaller pancakes work best, as being a gluten free recipe, the pancakes are very soft and light. When bubbles appear, turn them over to finish cooking.

LUNCH

Broccoli & Fennel Soup

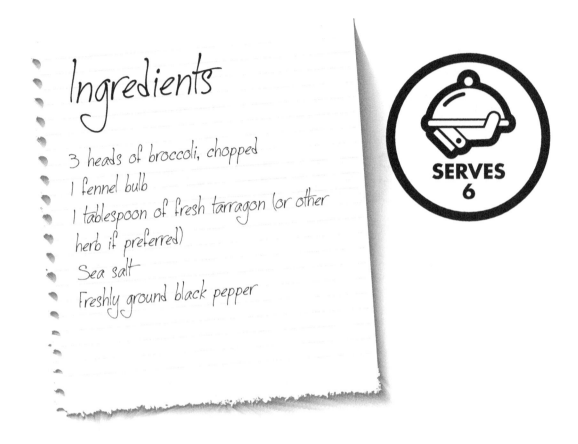

Ingredients

3 heads of broccoli, chopped
1 fennel bulb
1 tablespoon of fresh tarragon (or other herb if preferred)
Sea salt
Freshly ground black pepper

SERVES 6

Method

Place the broccoli and fennel in enough water to cover them and bring to the boil. Simmer for 7 minutes. When cooked, transfer to a food processor and blend until smooth. Add more water if required to adjust the consistency. Return the soup to the saucepan, add the tarragon and season with salt and pepper. Heat through before serving.

Butternut Squash & Ginger Soup

SERVES 4

Ingredients

1 tablespoon olive oil
1 medium onion, chopped
1 butternut squash, peeled, de-seeded and chopped
1 litre (1 ½ pints) of water or gluten-free vegetable stock (broth)
1 tablespoon fresh ginger, chopped
120ml (4fl oz or ½ cup) coconut milk

Method

Heat the oil in a saucepan. Add the onion and cook until soft. Add the squash, ginger and stock (broth) or water. Cook on a low to medium heat until the squash is soft. Stir in the coconut milk and heat thoroughly. Blend until smooth and serve.

Avocado & Melon Salad

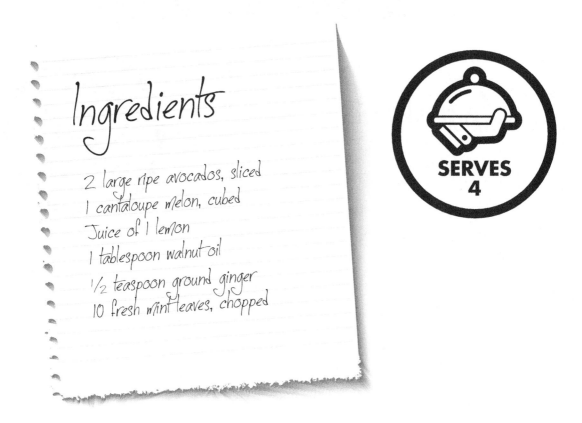

Ingredients

2 large ripe avocados, sliced
1 cantaloupe melon, cubed
Juice of 1 lemon
1 tablespoon walnut oil
½ teaspoon ground ginger
10 fresh mint leaves, chopped

SERVES
4

Method

Mix the walnut oil, lemon juice, ginger and mint leaves together in a bowl. Add the avocados and melon and toss gently. Marinate for 2-3 hours before serving.

Pear, Walnuts & Blue Cheese Salad

Ingredients

SERVES 2

2 pears, peeled
1 teaspoon olive oil
1 teaspoon butter
½ teaspoon ground coriander
125g (4oz) green salad leaves
25g (1oz) blue cheese, crumbled
2 tablespoon walnuts, roughly chopped
1 tablespoon lemon juice
Freshly ground black pepper

Method

Wash the pears and cut in half. Remove the core then cut each half into quarters. Heat the oil and butter in a pan. Add the pears and walnuts. Cook for 3 minutes until the pears are soft. Sprinkle with the ground coriander and pepper. Toss in a bowl with all the remaining ingredients. Serve immediately and enjoy.

Chicken & Sweetcorn Soup

Ingredients

1 tablespoon olive oil
1 chicken breast, chopped
1 clove of garlic, crushed
1 tablespoon cornflour (cornstarch)
600ml (1 pint) warm gluten-free chicken stock (broth)
100g (3 1/2 oz) sweetcorn kernels
1 egg
1 tablespoon lemon juice

SERVES 4

Method

Heat the oil in a saucepan. Add the chicken and garlic and cook gently for 3-4 minutes. In a cup, mix a tablespoon of cornflour (cornstarch) with a tablespoon of stock (broth). Add it to the pan with the remaining stock (broth). Add the sweetcorn and bring to the boil. Simmer for 6-7 minutes, stirring occasionally. In a bowl whisk the egg with the lemon juice. Slowly add it to the soup, stirring gently as threads of egg form. Cook for another 1-2 minutes. Serve and enjoy.

Creamy Cauliflower Soup

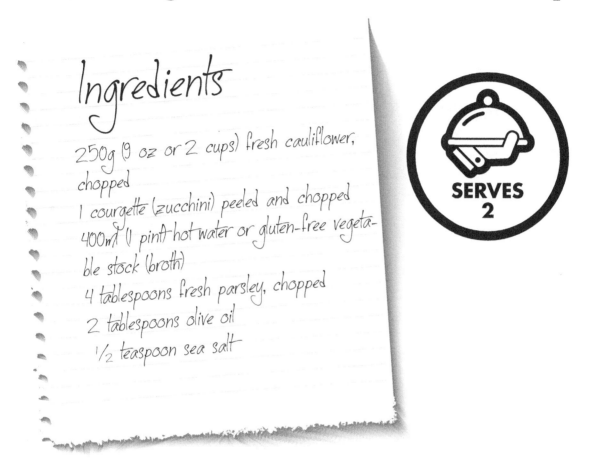

Ingredients

250g (9 oz or 2 cups) fresh cauliflower, chopped

1 courgette (zucchini) peeled and chopped

400ml (1 pint) hot water or gluten-free vegetable stock (broth)

4 tablespoons fresh parsley, chopped

2 tablespoons olive oil

½ teaspoon sea salt

SERVES 2

Method

Heat the olive oil in a large saucepan and add the cauliflower and courgette (zucchini). Cook for around 5 minutes, stirring occasionally. Add the water or stock, salt and water and simmer gently for 15 minutes. Pour the soup into a blender, add the parsley and blitz until smooth. Return the soup to the saucepan and gently simmer for 5 minutes or until heated through. Can be served either hot or cold.

Pumpkin Soup

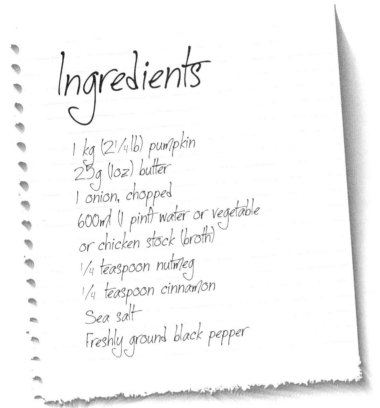

Ingredients

1 kg (2¼ lb) pumpkin
25g (1oz) butter
1 onion, chopped
600ml (1 pint) water or vegetable
or chicken stock (broth)
¼ teaspoon nutmeg
¼ teaspoon cinnamon
Sea salt
Freshly ground black pepper

SERVES
6-8

Method

Cut open the pumpkin, remove the seeds and discard. Cut the flesh into cubes. Heat the butter in a pan and add the onion. Cook until it becomes soft. Add to the pan the pumpkin and water or stock (broth). Bring to the boil, reduce the heat and simmer for 30 minutes. Transfer to a food processor or use a hand blender to make a puree from the soup. Return to the pan and add the nutmeg, cinnamon, salt and pepper.

Spicy Lentil Soup

Ingredients

175g (6oz) red lentils
1 litre (1 1/2 pints) water
1 bay leaf
2 tablespoons olive oil
1 clove of garlic, crushed
1 onion, chopped
2 carrots, chopped
2 sticks of celery, chopped
1 teaspoon ground coriander
1/2 teaspoon turmeric
1/2 teaspoon ground cumin
1/2 teaspoon chilli powder
Sea salt
Freshly ground black pepper

SERVES 6

Method

Heat the olive oil in a saucepan and add the cumin and onion. Cook for 5 minutes to soften the onion. Add the garlic, celery and carrots and cook for 10 minutes. Add all the remaining spices and cook for 2 minutes. Add the lentils then pour in the water. Bring to the boil, reduce the heat and simmer for 50 minutes. Remove the bay leaf then transfer the soup to a blender and process until smooth. Return the soup to the saucepan and heat thoroughly. Season and serve.

Chilli & Lime Chicken Strips

SERVES 4-6

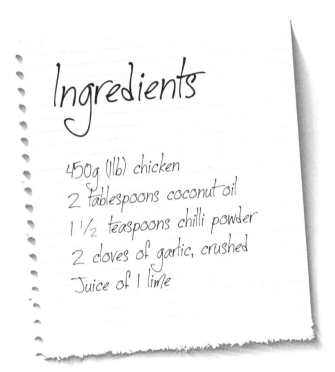

Ingredients

450g (1lb) chicken
2 tablespoons coconut oil
1 1/2 teaspoons chilli powder
2 cloves of garlic, crushed
Juice of 1 lime

Method

Slice the chicken into small strips. Heat the coconut oil in a frying pan over a medium heat and add the cicken. Stir-fry the strips for 2-3 minutes, then add the chilli powder, garlic and lime juice. Continue stirring for another 6-7 minutes or until cooked thoroughly. These strips are a great, versatile and tasty addition to many dishes. You can add them to salads, rice, stir fries and wraps. They can also be a handy high protein snack for lunch on the go.

Courgette (Zucchini) 'Spaghetti'

SERVES 2

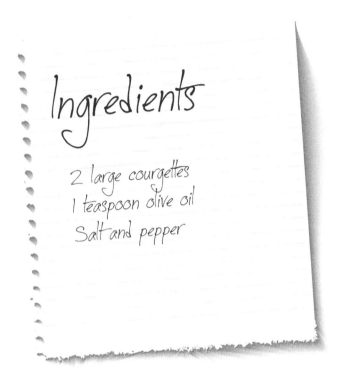

Ingredients

2 large courgettes
1 teaspoon olive oil
Salt and pepper

Method

Peel strips of courgette and cut them into 1cm (½ inch) wide strips or use a julienne peeler or spiralizer. Heat the olive oil in a frying pan. Add the courgette strips and cook for 2/3 minutes. Season with salt and pepper. Serve with tomato and herb sauce (see recipe at rear of book) as a great alternative to pasta.

Cauliflower 'Couscous'

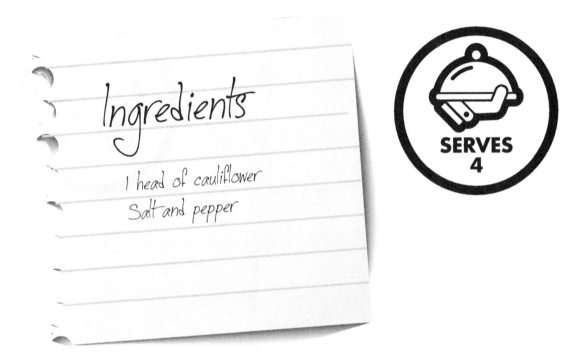

Ingredients

1 head of cauliflower
Salt and pepper

SERVES
4

Method

Grate (shred) the cauliflower by hand or use a food processor. Place the cauliflower in a saucepan of boiling water and cook for 6-8 minutes until the cauliflower is soft and tender. Serve immediately.

Quinoa Tabbouleh

Ingredients

120g (4oz or 2/3 cup) quinoa, cooked
75g (3oz or 1/2 cup) spring onions
(scallions), chopped
1 cucumber, peeled and diced
Juice of 1 lemon
1 tomato, diced
4 tablespoons fresh parsley, chopped
4 tablespoons fresh mint, chopped
1 tablespoon olive oil
Sea salt
Freshly ground black pepper

SERVES 4

Method

Combine all of the ingredients in a large bowl. Season with salt and pepper. Stir, cover and place it in the fridge for at least 30 minutes to chill before serving. Serve as a tasty, nutritious accompaniment to meat, chicken or fish.

Salad Nicoise

Ingredients

50g (2oz) tinned tuna, drained
2 new potatoes, cooked and quartered
50g (2oz) green beans, cooked
1 hard-boiled egg, peeled and quartered
4 black olives
25g (1oz) chopped lettuce
1 tablespoon mustard vinaigrette
1 tomato, quartered
1 anchovy fillet (optional)
1 tablespoon fresh parsley, chopped
Sea salt
Freshly ground black pepper

SERVES 1

Method

Put the green beans, potatoes and lettuce into a bowl. For the recipe for mustard vinaigrette, see the back of the book under sauces and condiments. Add the vinaigrette and toss the ingredients in it. Serve onto a plate and top with tuna, olives, tomato, egg and anchovy (optional). Season with salt and pepper and sprinkle with parsley.

Pesto Lamb Chops

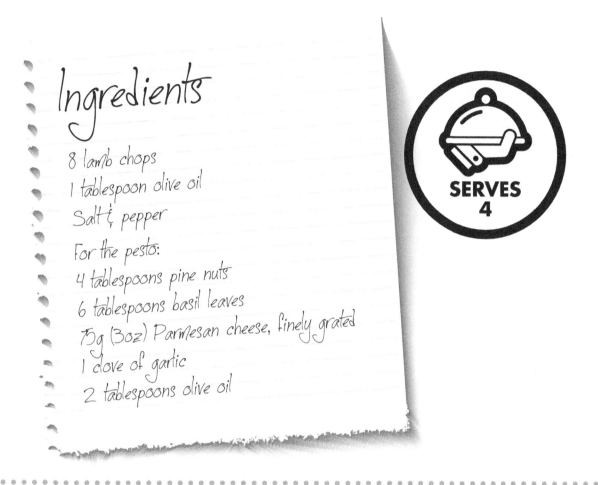

Ingredients

8 lamb chops
1 tablespoon olive oil
Salt & pepper

For the pesto:
4 tablespoons pine nuts
6 tablespoons basil leaves
75g (3oz) Parmesan cheese, finely grated
1 clove of garlic
2 tablespoons olive oil

SERVES 4

Method

For the pesto; put all of the ingredients into a blender and blitz until you have a smooth paste. Set it aside.

For the chops; season them with salt and pepper. Heat the oil in a pan and fry the chops for 2-3 minutes on each side, or longer if you like them well done. Transfer to a plate and cover with pesto. Serve alongside a green salad and new potatoes.

Curry Butter Chicken

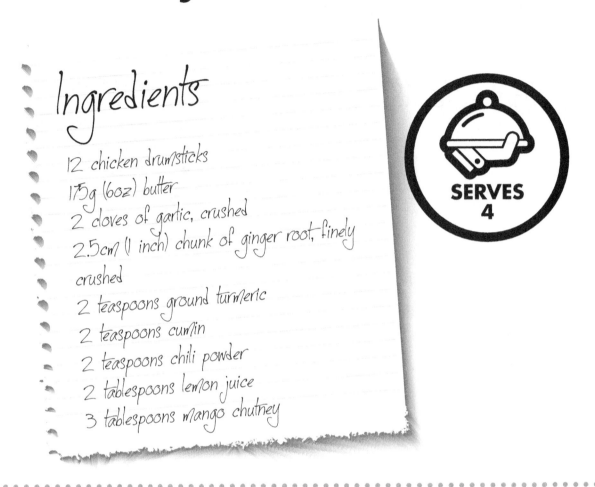

Ingredients

12 chicken drumsticks
175g (6oz) butter
2 cloves of garlic, crushed
2.5cm (1 inch) chunk of ginger root, finely crushed
2 teaspoons ground turmeric
2 teaspoons cumin
2 teaspoons chili powder
2 tablespoons lemon juice
3 tablespoons mango chutney

SERVES 4

Method

Put the butter, garlic, ginger, cumin, turmeric, chilli powder, lemon juice and mango chutney into a bowl and mix until it is well blended. Make 3 incisions in each chicken drumstick. Grill (broil) the chicken for around 12 minutes, turning ½ way through. Remove them and thickly spread curry butter onto each piece of chicken, getting plenty of the mixture into the incisions. Grill (broil) for another 5 minutes, basting them with the curry butter. They can be served hot or cold.

Peanut & Sesame Chicken

Ingredients

2 tablespoons olive oil

2 tablespoons sesame oil

4 chicken breasts, sliced

250g (9 oz) broccoli, broken into florets

250g (9 oz) baby corn

1 red (bell) pepper, chopped

2 tablespoons tamari sauce (gluten-free)

250ml (8fl oz) orange juice

2 teaspoons cornflour (corn starch)

2 tablespoons toasted sesame seeds

60g (2 ½ oz) unsalted peanuts

SERVES 4

Method

Heat both of the oils in a large frying pan. Add the chicken and cook for 4-5 minutes. Add in the broccoli, red pepper and baby corn. Stir and cook for 2 minutes. In a separate bowl mix the tamari, orange juice and cornflour. Pour it into the pan with the chicken and vegetables. The sauce will thicken and form a glaze. Sprinkle on the peanuts and sesame seeds and warm them through. Serve with rice noodles or rice.

Potato Skins

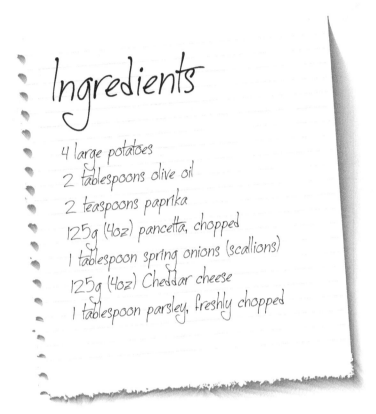

Ingredients

4 large potatoes
2 tablespoons olive oil
2 teaspoons paprika
125g (4oz) pancetta, chopped
1 tablespoon spring onions (scallions)
125g (4oz) Cheddar cheese
1 tablespoon parsley, freshly chopped

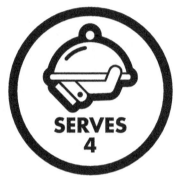

SERVES
4

Method

Preheat the oven to 200C/400F. Prick potatoes with a fork and place them on the top shelf of the oven. Bake for an hour or until soft right through. Leave the potatoes to cool. Cut in half and scoop the flesh into a bowl and set aside. Combine the oil and paprika and use some of it to brush the outside of the potato skins. Place under a hot grill for 5 minutes, until crisp, turning occasionally. Heat the remaining oil and paprika and fry the pancetta until it's crispy. Add this to the potato flesh, along with the spring onions (scallions), cheese and parsley. Mix well. Fill the potato skins with the mixture. Place the skins in the oven for a further 15 minutes, making sure they are heated thoroughly.

Gluten-Free Baked Beans

Ingredients

2 x 400g (2 x 14oz) tins of cannellini beans, rinsed and drained

1 x 400g (14oz) tin of chopped tomatoes

1 onion, peeled and very finely chopped

1 clove garlic, crushed

1 teaspoon smoked paprika

1 large sprig rosemary

1/2 teaspoon cinnamon

1/4 teaspoon nutmeg (optional)

1 tablespoon olive oil

Splash of Worcestershire sauce (double check it's gluten-free)

Sea salt, Freshly ground black pepper

SERVES 4

Method

Heat the oil in a frying pan and add the onion, garlic and rosemary. Fry for 4-5 minutes, until the onion is soft. Add the smoked paprika, cinnamon and nutmeg (if desired) and stir. Add the cannellini beans and tomatoes. Reduce the heat and simmer for around 20 minutes. You may need to add a little water. Add a splash of Worcestershire sauce and season with salt and pepper. Simmer for another few minutes to reduce down. Remove the rosemary sprig and serve.

Thai Chicken Burgers

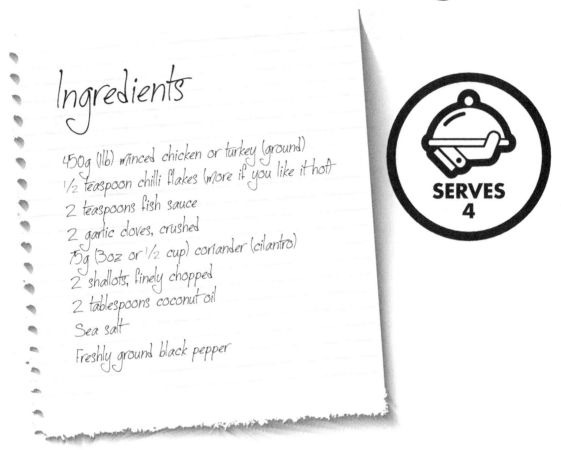

Ingredients

450g (1lb) minced chicken or turkey (ground)
½ teaspoon chilli flakes (more if you like it hot)
2 teaspoons fish sauce
2 garlic cloves, crushed
75g (3oz or ½ cup) coriander (cilantro)
2 shallots, finely chopped
2 tablespoons coconut oil
Sea salt
Freshly ground black pepper

SERVES 4

Method

Place the chicken or turkey in a large bowl and add the coriander (cilantro), fish sauce, garlic, shallots and chilli flakes. Season with salt and pepper. Mix the ingredients together well. Divide the mixture into 4 and form into burger shapes. Heat the coconut oil in a frying pan. Place the burgers in the pan and cook for around 7- 8 minutes on either side until the burgers are cooked through. Serve them in iceberg or romaine lettuce leaves instead of a bread bun.

Cauliflower Hash Browns

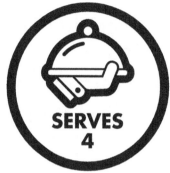

SERVES 4

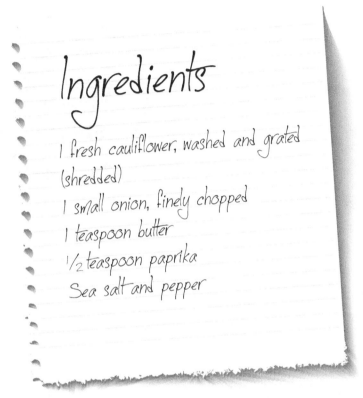

Ingredients

1 fresh cauliflower, washed and grated (shredded)
1 small onion, finely chopped
1 teaspoon butter
1/2 teaspoon paprika
Sea salt and pepper

Method

Heat the butter in a frying pan and add the onion. Cook until the onion becomes soft. Add the grated cauliflower. Stir and cook until the cauliflower is tender and golden brown. Add some extra butter if you need to. Season with paprika, salt and pepper and serve.

Quick Italian Chicken

Ingredients

250g (9 oz) chicken, cooked and chopped
(leftovers are perfect)
250g (9 oz) mushrooms, chopped
1 onion, chopped
1 x 400g (14oz) can of chopped tomatoes
2 cloves of garlic
1 tablespoon olive oil
1 tablespoon fresh oregano, chopped
1 tablespoon fresh basil, chopped

**SERVES
2**

Method

Heat the olive oil in a pan. Add the onion and mushrooms. Cook until the onion has softened. Stir in the tomatoes, garlic, basil and oregano. Simmer for 5 minutes. Add the chicken and heat through for 2-3 minutes. Serve and enjoy.

DINNER

Garlic & Herb Chicken

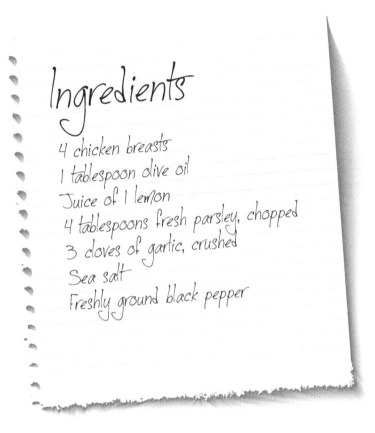

Ingredients

4 chicken breasts
1 tablespoon olive oil
Juice of 1 lemon
4 tablespoons fresh parsley, chopped
3 cloves of garlic, crushed
Sea salt
Freshly ground black pepper

SERVES
4

Method

In a bowl, place the olive oil, parsley, lemon juice and garlic. Add the chicken and coat it with the mixture. Place in the fridge and marinate for 30 minutes, or longer if possible. When you're ready to cook the chicken, heat a little olive oil in a pan. Place the chicken in the pan cook for around 5 minutes on each side or until the chicken is thoroughly cooked. Season and serve with salad or vegetables.

Shepherd's Pie

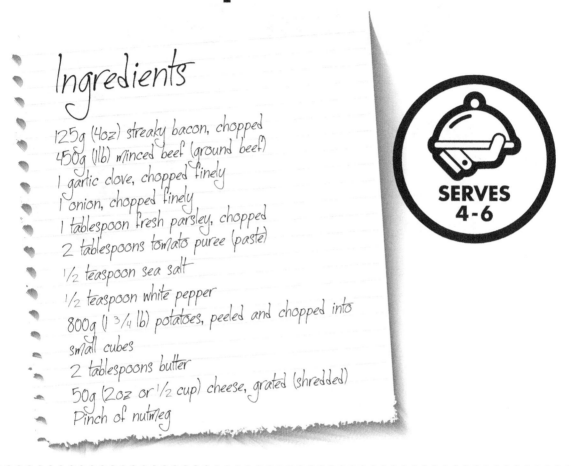

Ingredients

125g (4oz) streaky bacon, chopped
450g (1lb) minced beef (ground beef)
1 garlic clove, chopped finely
1 onion, chopped finely
1 tablespoon fresh parsley, chopped
2 tablespoons tomato puree (paste)
1/2 teaspoon sea salt
1/2 teaspoon white pepper
800g (1 3/4 lb) potatoes, peeled and chopped into small cubes
2 tablespoons butter
50g (2oz or 1/2 cup) cheese, grated (shredded)
Pinch of nutmeg

SERVES 4-6

Method

In a large pan, fry the bacon until crispy and set aside. Add the beef to the frying pan and cook for 2 minutes. Add the garlic, onion, tomato paste, parsley, salt and pepper. Cover and cook on a low heat for 30 minutes, stirring occasionally. Meanwhile, boil the potatoes for around 10 minutes or until tender. Drain them, add the butter, nutmeg and mash them. Preheat the oven to 230C/450F. Spread the beef mixture onto the bottom of an ovenproof casserole dish. Add the mashed potato layer on top and smooth out with the back of a spoon. Sprinkle with cheese and bake in the oven for around 20 minutes or until the pie is lightly browned and the cheese melted.

Tomato & Aubergine (Eggplant) Gratin

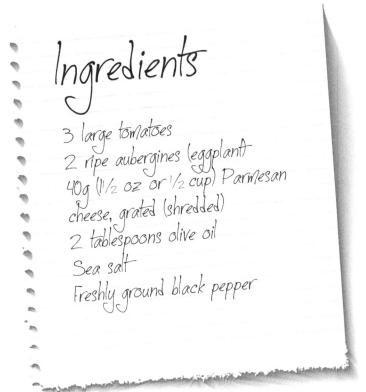

Ingredients

3 large tomatoes
2 ripe aubergines (eggplant)
40g (1½ oz or ½ cup) Parmesan
cheese, grated (shredded)
2 tablespoons olive oil
Sea salt
Freshly ground black pepper

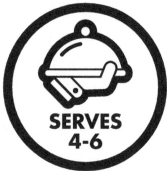

SERVES
4-6

Method

Cut the tomatoes into slices and set aside. Thinly slice the aubergines (eggplants) and place on a grill rack lined with foil. Brush with olive oil and grill (broil) for 15 minutes, turning once until golden on both sides. Place the tomato slices and aubergine slices in an oven-proof dish, alternating between slices of each. Cover with the grated Parmesan and season with salt and pepper. Transfer to the oven and bake at 200C/400F for 15 minutes, or until the cheese is golden. Serve and eat immediately.

Gluten-Free Pizza

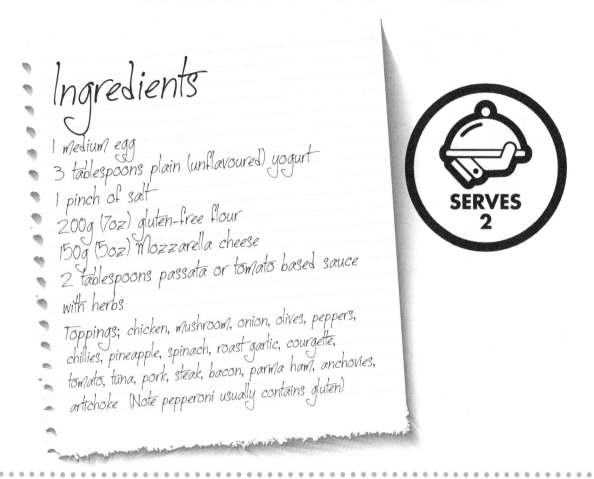

Ingredients

1 medium egg
3 tablespoons plain (unflavoured) yogurt
1 pinch of salt
200g (7oz) gluten-free flour
150g (5oz) Mozzarella cheese
2 tablespoons passata or tomato based sauce
with herbs
Toppings; chicken, mushroom, onion, olives, peppers,
chillies, pineapple, spinach, roast garlic, courgette,
tomato, tuna, pork, steak, bacon, parma ham, anchovies,
artichoke (Note pepperoni usually contains gluten)

SERVES 2

Method

In a bowl beat the egg and combine with the yogurt. Add a pinch of salt and stir. Gradually add the flour a little at a time, using a knife or a food mixer until it starts to become doughy. Use your hands and keep adding the flour. Knead the dough until it becomes soft but not sticky. Very lightly grease a baking tray. Use either your palms or a rolling pin to flatten the dough to between ½ cm and 1½ cm depending on how thick you like your pizza. Prick the base all over using a fork.

Spread on the tomato based sauce. Less is more to prevent it being soggy. Add mozzarella cheese and your favourite topping. Place it in the oven at 200C/400F for 15-20 minutes until the cheese has melted and the crust is golden. Serve and enjoy.

Lamb Steaks With Mango & Tomato Salsa

SERVES 4

Ingredients

- 4 lamb steaks
- 1 tablespoon fresh rosemary leaves, chopped
- 3 cloves of garlic, crushed
- 4 tablespoons olive oil
- 4 tomatoes, seeds removed and chopped
- 100g (3½ oz) mango, peeled and chopped
- 1 teaspoon fresh chives, chopped
- Sea salt
- Freshly ground black pepper

Method

Combine the rosemary, 2 cloves of crushed garlic and 3 teaspoons of olive oil and coat the lamb with the mixture. Season with salt and pepper. Cover, chill and marinate for 1 hour or overnight is even better. When you are ready to cook them, place the marinated steaks under a hot grill for 3-5 minutes on each side depending on how you like it. Meanwhile to make the salsa, mix the tomatoes, chives, mango, 1 clove of crushed garlic and a tablespoon of olive oil in a bowl. When the lamb is ready, serve it with a spoonful of the salsa on top.

Celeriac & Apple Mash

Ingredients

- 1 celeriac
- 1 apple
- 25g (1oz) butter
- Sea salt & black pepper

SERVES
4

Method

Peel and core the apple and cut into chunks. Peel the celeriac and chop it into chunks. Place both the apple and celeriac in a saucepan, cover it with boiling water. Simmer for 20 minutes. Drain the apple and celeriac, add the butter and mash it. Season and serve with rich meat dishes.

Sweet Potato & Spring Onion Mash

Ingredients

- 700g (1lb 9 oz) sweet potato, peeled and chopped
- 1 bunch of spring onions (scallion), finely chopped
- ½ teaspoon ground nutmeg
- 2 teaspoons butter

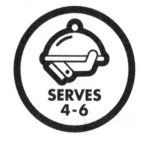

SERVES
4-6

Method

Place the sweet potatoes in a saucepan, bring to the boil and simmer for 10-12 minutes, until soft. Drain the sweet potatoes but leave them in the saucepan. Add the spring onions, nutmeg and butter. Mash until the sweet potatoes is smooth. Season and serve.

Thai Green Curry Vegetables

Ingredients

2 tablespoons coconut oil
100g (3oz) green beans, sliced lengthways
1 red pepper (Bell pepper), chopped
1 green pepper (Bell pepper), chopped
1 onion, chopped
1 bunch spring onions (scallions), chopped
1 medium carrot, chopped
3 teaspoons Thai green curry paste
400ml (14fl oz) coconut milk
2 tablespoons fresh coriander leaves (cilantro), chopped
Extra coriander to garnish (optional)

SERVES 4-6

Method

Heat the coconut oil in a large pan. Add the onion and carrots and fry for 5 minutes. Add the remaining vegetables and cook for a further 3 minutes. Add the curry paste and coconut milk. Cover and simmer for 10 minutes until the vegetables are tender but firm. Add the chopped coriander (cilantro) and stir. Transfer to serving bowls and sprinkle with a little extra coriander.

Mexican Bean Burgers

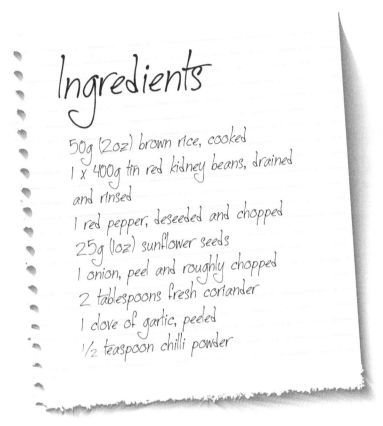

Ingredients

50g (2oz) brown rice, cooked
1 x 400g tin red kidney beans, drained
and rinsed
1 red pepper, deseeded and chopped
25g (1oz) sunflower seeds
1 onion, peel and roughly chopped
2 tablespoons fresh coriander
1 clove of garlic, peeled
1/2 teaspoon chilli powder

SERVES 4

Method

Place in a food processor the beans, garlic, onion, pepper, sunflower seeds, coriander, chilli powder and brown rice. Blend for a short time only, until the mixture is thick but not smooth. Scoop it out and place it in a bowl. Transfer to the fridge to chill for 20-30 minutes. Lightly grease a baking tray and preheat the oven to 200C/400F. Remove the mixture from the fridge and mould it into 8 patties. Bake for 20-25 minutes until golden brown. Serve with guacamole or tomato salsa and salad.

Spinach & Mushroom Crustless Quiche

Ingredients

225g (8oz) fresh mushrooms, sliced
1 garlic clove, crushed
1/2 tablespoon olive oil
100g (3 1/2 oz) fresh spinach leaves
4 eggs
200ml (7fl oz or 1 cup) milk
40g (1 1/2 oz) feta cheese, crumbled
40g (1 1/2 oz) grated (shredded) mozzarella cheese
Sea salt
Freshly ground black pepper

SERVES 4-6

Method

Heat the olive oil in a pan. Add the mushrooms, spinach, garlic and season with salt and pepper. Cook until the mushrooms have softened. Grease a pie dish. Add the cooked mushrooms mixture and the feta cheese. In a bowl, whisk the eggs and add the milk. Pour this mixture into the pie dish over the spinach, mushrooms, and feta. Sprinkle the top with mozzarella cheese. Place it on a baking sheet and transfer to the oven. Bake in the oven at 180C/350F for 45 minutes, or until it is golden brown and completely set. Remove, slice and serve.

Bacon & Broccoli Hash

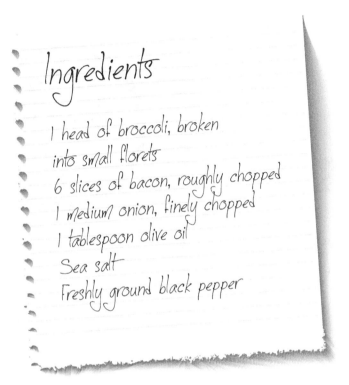

Ingredients

1 head of broccoli, broken
into small florets
6 slices of bacon, roughly chopped
1 medium onion, finely chopped
1 tablespoon olive oil
Sea salt
Freshly ground black pepper

SERVES 4

Method

Steam the broccoli in a steamer for 4 minutes. Heat the olive oil in a frying pan. Add the bacon and onion. Fry until the bacon is cooked. Add the broccoli to the pan and stir. Cook for around 10 minutes until it becomes crispy. Alternatively you use left-over vegetables like potatoes, turnip and carrot in place of, or as well as the broccoli.

Stuffed Peppers

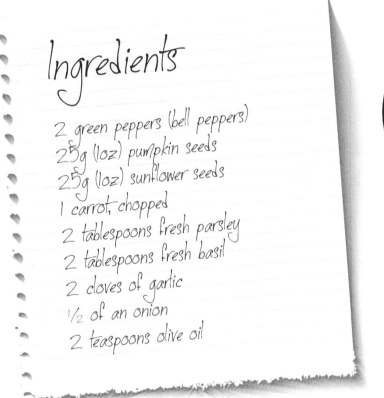

Ingredients

2 green peppers (bell peppers)
25g (1oz) pumpkin seeds
25g (1oz) sunflower seeds
1 carrot, chopped
2 tablespoons fresh parsley
2 tablespoons fresh basil
2 cloves of garlic
½ of an onion
2 teaspoons olive oil

SERVES 2

Method

Put the carrot, seeds, garlic, herbs, olive oil and onion into a blender and blitz until it is well combined. Cut the peppers in half and remove and discard the seeds. Stuff the peppers with the seed mixture. Place on a baking sheet, transfer to the oven and bake at 180C/350F for 20 minutes.

Roast Chicken, Chickpeas & Squash

Ingredients

2 red onions, cut into wedges
600g (1lb 5oz) sweet potato peeled and chopped
4 tomatoes, halved
2 garlic cloves, thinly sliced
2 tablespoons olive oil
8 chicken thigh fillets
200g (7oz) chickpeas
4 tablespoons fresh parsley, chopped
Sea salt
Freshly ground black pepper

SERVES
4

Method

Preheat oven to 220C/425F. Combine the onion, sweet potato, tomato, garlic and half the oil in a bowl. Transfer to large baking tray. Bake for 15 minutes. Meanwhile, heat the remaining oil in a frying pan. Season the chicken with salt and pepper. Cook for 2-3 minutes each side or until golden. Add the chicken to the tray and bake for a further 10 minutes or until the chicken is cooked through. Add the chickpeas, parsley and stir. Heat thoroughly and serve.

Lamb Kebabs & Coriander Dip

Ingredients

150g (5oz) natural yogurt (unflavoured)
450g (1lb) boneless lamb, cut into chunks
1 teaspoon ground coriander
1 teaspoon ground cumin
Juice of 1/2 a lemon

Coriander Raita:
3 tablespoons fresh coriander, chopped
250g (9 oz) natural yogurt
(unflavoured)

**SERVES
4**

Method

Chop the lamb into bite-size chunks. In a bowl, combine 150g (5oz) yogurt, cumin, coriander (cilantro) and lemon juice. Add the lamb to the marinade, cover and place in the fridge for one hour. (It's even better if you can leave it overnight). Meanwhile to make the dip, combine the yogurt and fresh coriander then place it in the fridge to chill. Once the lamb is marinated, thread the lamb chunks onto skewers. Place under a hot grill (broiler) for 5 minutes on either side. Serve with the coriander dip.

Prawns & Scallops with Tangy Dressing

Ingredients

16 large raw prawns (shrimp), shelled
24 fresh scallops
1 ripe mango, peeled, stoned and cut into chunks
125g (4oz) green salad leaves
1 tablespoon olive oil

For the dressing:
Juice of ½ grapefruit
Juice and rind from 1 lemon
1 teaspoon honey
5 tablespoons olive oil

SERVES 4

Method

For the dressing; place all the ingredients in a bowl and mix. Add the prawns (shrimps), scallops and mango to the dressing and coat them completely. Thread them onto skewers. Heat a tablespoon of oil in a frying pan and add the prawn and scallop skewers. Cook for 6-7 minutes, turning to make sure everything cooks thoroughly, evenly and golden brown. Serve onto plates alongside the salad and drizzle over the tangy citrus dressing.

Sweet Potato Balls

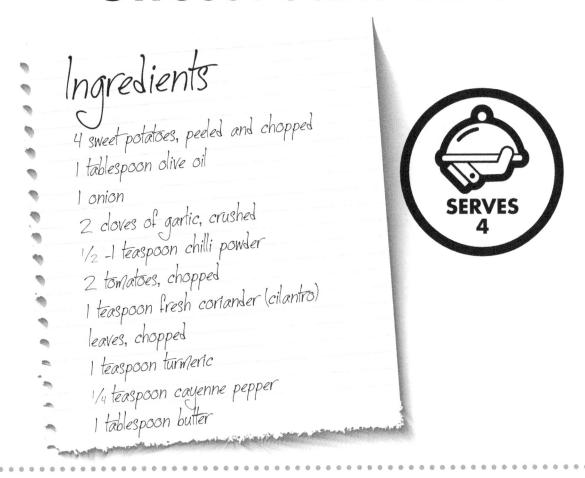

Ingredients

4 sweet potatoes, peeled and chopped
1 tablespoon olive oil
1 onion
2 cloves of garlic, crushed
½ –1 teaspoon chilli powder
2 tomatoes, chopped
1 teaspoon fresh coriander (cilantro)
leaves, chopped
1 teaspoon turmeric
¼ teaspoon cayenne pepper
1 tablespoon butter

SERVES
4

Method

Preheat the oven to 180C/350F. Steam or boil the sweet potatoes until they are soft. Mash them with the butter. Heat the olive oil in a frying pan. Add the onion, garlic and chilli powder. Cook until the onion is soft. Add the coriander (cilantro), tomatoes and spice. Stir well. Add the onion and tomato mixture to the mashed sweet potato and combine. Using your hands, form the mixture into balls and place them on a baking tray. Bake in the oven for 15-20 minutes. Serve and enjoy.

Chicken Satay Skewers

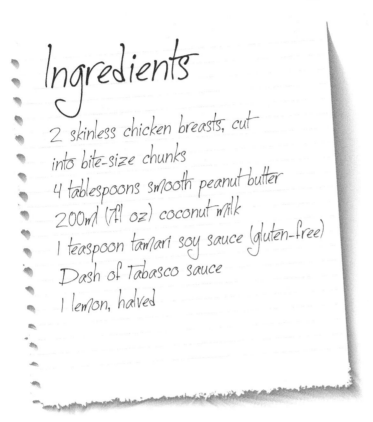

Ingredients

2 skinless chicken breasts, cut into bite-size chunks
4 tablespoons smooth peanut butter
200ml (7fl oz) coconut milk
1 teaspoon tamari soy sauce (gluten-free)
Dash of Tabasco sauce
1 lemon, halved

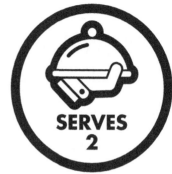

SERVES
2

Method

Preheat the oven to 200C/400F. Put the peanut butter and coconut milk into a bowl. Mix well. Add the Tabasco, tamari sauce and stir. Place the chicken chunks in a bowl and pour the peanut sauce over it. Coat the chicken completely. Thread the chicken onto skewers, and set aside the remaining satay sauce. Place the chicken skewers under a hot grill (broiler) and cook for 4-5 minutes on each side, making sure it's cooked through. Place the remaining satay sauce in a small pan and add the juice from half a lemon. Heat it thoroughly. Cut the remaining lemon into 2 wedges. Serve the chicken skewers and pour the remaining satay sauce on top. Place the lemon garnish on the side.

Rice Cubes & Coriander Dipping Sauce

SERVES 4-6

Ingredients

300g (11oz or 1 1/2 cups) thai jasmine rice, cooked

For coriander dip

2 cloves of garlic

2 tablespoons peanut butter

3 tablespoons lemon juice

175ml (6fl oz or   cup) coconut milk

2 spring onions (scallions), chopped

1 tablespoon ground black pepper

60g (2oz or 1 cup) fresh coriander

1 red chilli, deseeded and chopped

Method

Grease and line a 20 x 10 cm (8 x 4 inch) tin. Put half the cooked jasmine rice into a blender and process until smooth. Mix the blended rice with the remaining rice. Scoop and compress it into the tin. Cover with cling film (plastic wrap). Place a chopping board on top to weigh it down. Chill overnight. When you are ready, remove the film, sprinkle with a tablespoon of water. Cover with foil and warm in the oven at 180/350F for around 10-15 minutes. Put the coriander, garlic, pepper, peanut butter, spring onions, coconut milk, chilli and lemon juice into a blender and blitz until smooth. Transfer to a saucepan and heat thoroughly. Remove the rice from the oven and cut it into cubes. Serve with the coriander dipping sauce.

Polenta Chips

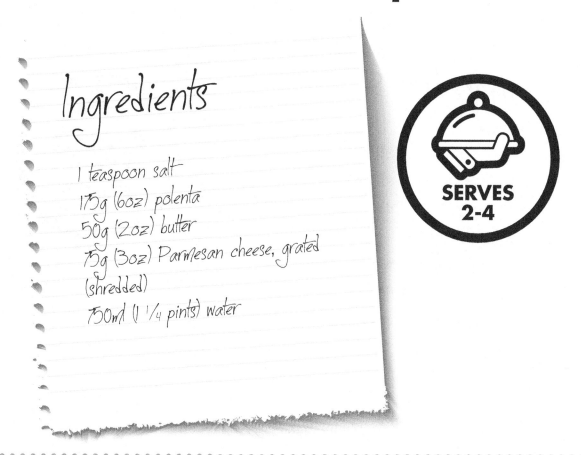

Ingredients

1 teaspoon salt
175g (6oz) polenta
50g (2oz) butter
75g (3oz) Parmesan cheese, grated (shredded)
750ml (1 ¼ pints) water

SERVES 2-4

Method

Bring the water to the boil and add the salt. Slowly and steadily add the polenta, stirring to prevent lumps from forming. Reduce the heat and simmer while stirring continuously. The polenta will thicken very quickly, in around a minute. When it does, turn off the heat. Now add the butter and Parmesan and combine. Tip the mixture into a baking dish of about 2cm (1 inch) in depth. Smooth it out. Leave it to cool for about 30 minutes or until it is set. Cut the polenta into strips, resembling chips (fries). Lay them out on a baking sheet and bake at 220C/425F for 15-20 minutes or until they are firm and easily lift off the baking tray. Serve and enjoy.

Roast Lemon Chilli Chicken

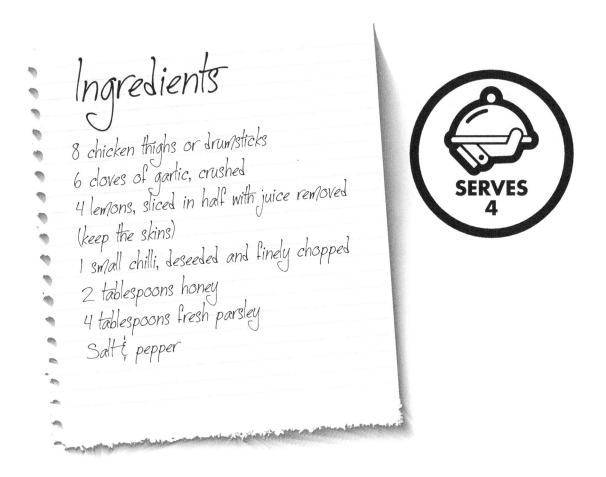

Ingredients

8 chicken thighs or drumsticks
6 cloves of garlic, crushed
4 lemons, sliced in half with juice removed
(keep the skins)
1 small chilli, deseeded and finely chopped
2 tablespoons honey
4 tablespoons fresh parsley
Salt & pepper

SERVES 4

Method

Place the chicken in a casserole dish. In a bowl place the lemon juice, chilli, garlic and honey. Mix it well. Pour the juice over the chicken. Put the lemon skins into the casserole dish next to the chicken and marinate for at least 1 hour (overnight is even better). To cook the chicken, transfer it to the oven and cook at 200C/400F for around 45 minutes or until it's cooked thoroughly. Sprinkle with parsley and season with salt and pepper. Serve with rice, quinoa or salad.

Prosciutto Wrapped Prawns (Shrimps)

Ingredients

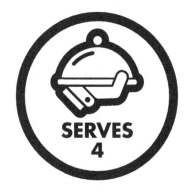

SERVES
4

20 large peeled, deveined, prawns (shrimps)
1 tablespoon fresh basil, chopped
1 teaspoon olive oil
1/2 teaspoon lemon zest
1/2 teaspoon sea salt
1/4 teaspoon chilli flakes
1/8 teaspoon freshly ground black pepper
10 slices prosciutto
1 lemon, quartered for garnish

Method

In a medium bowl, combine the prawns, basil, olive oil, zest, salt, chilli flakes, and black pepper. Mix well and set aside. Lay out the prosciutto in slices, and cut it in half length-wise so you have 20 pieces. Wrap the prosciutto around each shrimp then thread onto a skewer. Repeat for the remaining prawns and place 5 prawns on each skewer. Place the skewers under a grill (broiler) and cook for around 2 minutes on each side. Serve hot with lemon wedges.

Chunky Vegetarian Chilli

Ingredients

- 1 tablespoon olive oil
- 1 large onion, chopped
- 1 red pepper (bell pepper) chopped
- 1 green pepper (bell pepper) chopped
- 2 cloves of garlic, crushed
- 1 1/2 teaspoon lemon zest
- 1/2 teaspoons chilli powder
- 1 teaspoon ground cumin
- 1 teaspoon dried oregano
- 1/2 teaspoon lemon zest
- 1/2 teaspoon salt
- 1/2 teaspoon lemon zest
- 1/2 teaspoon black pepper
- 2 x 400g (14 oz) tins of chopped tomatoes
- 2 x 400g (14 oz) tins black beans
- 1 x 400g (14 oz) tin kidney beans

SERVES 6

Method

Heat the oil in a saucepan. Add the onion, bell peppers, and garlic and fry for 5 minutes or until tender. Add the remaining ingredients, and bring to a boil. Reduce heat, and simmer 30 minutes. Serve with rice. This recipe also works well in a slow cooker. Instead of simmering for 30 minutes, transfer it to a slow cooker, cook on a medium heat and it can be ready when you want it.

Orange Pork & Leeks

Ingredients

4 pork chops
2 large leeks, thinly sliced
1 red pepper (bell pepper) sliced
150ml (5fl oz) gluten-free chicken stock (broth)
3 tablespoons orange juice (fresh or concentrated)
3 garlic cloves, crushed
1 tablespoon mustard (double check that it's gluten-free)
1/2 teaspoon paprika
1/4 teaspoon salt
1/4 teaspoon freshly ground black pepper
2 teaspoons olive oil

SERVES
4

Method

Sprinkle the pork chops with salt, and black pepper. Heat the oil in a frying pan. Add the pork and fry for 3 minutes on each side or until done. Remove the pork and keep it warm. Add to the pan the leeks, pepper (bell pepper), and garlic. Fry for 3 minutes until the leek has softened. Add in the stock (broth) orange juice, mustard, and paprika. Stir and cook for 2-3 minutes or until the liquid thickens slightly. Return the pork chops to the pan and coat it in the juices. Serve and enjoy.

Cheesy Sweet Potatoes

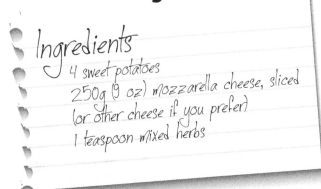

Ingredients
- 4 sweet potatoes
- 250g (9 oz) mozzarella cheese, sliced (or other cheese if you prefer)
- 1 teaspoon mixed herbs

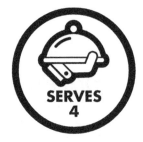

SERVES
4

Method

Prick the sweet potatoes with a fork. Place them in a pre-heated oven at 220C/425F for 40 minutes, or until they are soft. Remove and allow to cool slightly. Cut them in half, sprinkle with herbs and add a layer of sliced mozzarella. Place under a hot grill (broiler) until the cheese melts.

Salmon Burgers

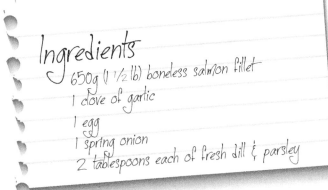

Ingredients
- 650g (1 1/2 lb) boneless salmon fillet
- 1 clove of garlic
- 1 egg
- 1 spring onion
- 2 tablespoons each of fresh dill & parsley

SERVES
6

Method

Put the salmon, spring onion, dill, parsley and garlic in a food processor. Blend until smooth. Place the mixture in a medium bowl and combine with the egg. Shape the mixture into patties. Cook under a hot grill (broiler) for 15 minutes, turning once halfway through.

Pumpkin Risotto

Ingredients

50g (2oz) butter
175g (6oz) onion, finely chopped
900g (2lb) pumpkin, peeled, de-seeded and cubed
2 cloves of garlic, crushed
225g (8oz) risotto rice (Arborio)
600ml (1pint) warm gluten-free chicken stock (broth)
40g (1 1/2 oz) Parmesan cheese, grated
Sea salt
Freshly ground black pepper

SERVES
6

Method

Melt the butter in a saucepan. Add the pumpkin and onion and gently fry until soft. Add the garlic and rice then mix well. Add in the stock (broth) a little at a time. Allow the rice to absorb most of the liquid before you add more. It will take around 20-25 minutes. Season it with salt and pepper. Sprinkle with parmesan cheese and stir. Serve and enjoy.

Lemon Risotto

Ingredients

1 tablespoon butter
1 onion, finely chopped
Zest and juice of 1 lemon
3 tablespoons olive oil
2 cloves of garlic, crushed
225g (8oz) risotto rice (Arborio)
600ml (1pint) warm gluten-free chicken stock (broth)
40g (1½ oz) Parmesan cheese, grated
200ml (7fl oz) dry white wine
3 tablespoons pine nuts
1 tablespoon fresh parsley, chopped
Sea salt & freshly ground black pepper

SERVES 4

Method

Heat the butter and oil in a pan. Add the onion and garlic and cook until the onion is soft. Add the rice and stir. Add the white wine, lemon juice and zest. Mix it together. Add in the stock (broth) a little at a time until the rice absorbs all of it. It should take around 20 minutes. Once the rice is soft and creamy, add in the pine nuts, Parmesan and parsley. Season with salt and pepper and serve.

Beef Stew

Ingredients

- 25g (1oz) cornflour
- 900g (2lb) stewing beef (chuck steak)
- 5 tablespoon olive oil
- 225g (8oz) mushrooms
- 225g (8oz) onion, finely chopped
- 4 cloves of garlic, crushed
- 2 tablespoons tomato puree
- 60ml (2fl oz) red wine vinegar (optional)
- 4 tablespoons fresh thyme, chopped
- 4 bay leaves
- 1 tablespoon freshly ground black pepper
- 5 whole cloves
- 900ml (1½ pints) gluten-free beef stock (broth)
- 900g (2lb) mixed root veg; parsnip, carrot, celeri-ac and turnip)
- Salt and pepper

SERVES 8

Method

Sprinkle the cornflour on a plate and coat the meat with it. Heat the olive oil in a flameproof casserole dish, add the meat and brown it for a few minutes. Add the tomato puree, garlic, vinegar, thyme, bay leaves, pepper and cloves and stock (broth). Stir and cook for 2-3 minutes. Add in the vegetables and bring to the boil. Season with salt and pepper. Transfer it to the oven and cook at 180C/350F for 1½ to 2 hours, until the meat is tender. Alternatively you can use a slow cooker for this.

Chicken Tagine

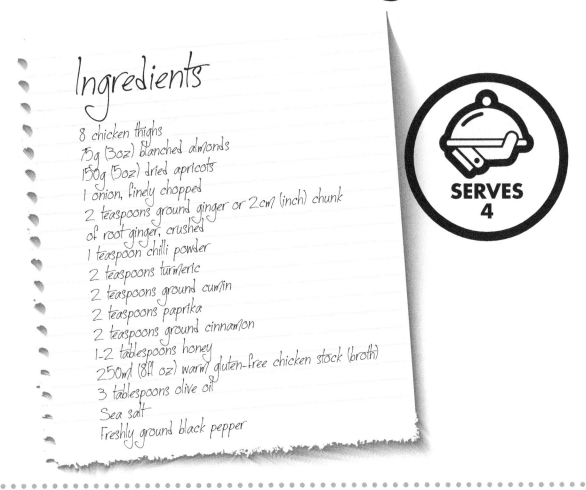

Ingredients

8 chicken thighs
75g (3oz) blanched almonds
150g (5oz) dried apricots
1 onion, finely chopped
2 teaspoons ground ginger or 2cm (inch) chunk
of root ginger, crushed
1 teaspoon chilli powder
2 teaspoons turmeric
2 teaspoons ground cumin
2 teaspoons paprika
2 teaspoons ground cinnamon
1-2 tablespoons honey
250ml (8fl oz) warm gluten-free chicken stock (broth)
3 tablespoons olive oil
Sea salt
Freshly ground black pepper

SERVES 4

Method

Heat 1 tablespoon of oil in a saucepan. Add the chicken and brown it for around 5 minutes. Remove and set aside. Add the remaining oil and the onion. Cook until softened. Add the ginger, chilli, turmeric, cumin, paprika and cinnamon and stir well. Return the chicken to the dish. Add the apricots, honey, chicken stock (broth) and almonds. Season with salt and pepper. Reduce the heat and simmer for 45 minutes until the chicken is tender. Serve with a garnish of flaked almonds. Tagine is traditionally served with couscous but it goes equally well with quinoa, which is gluten-free.

Cashew Crust Chicken

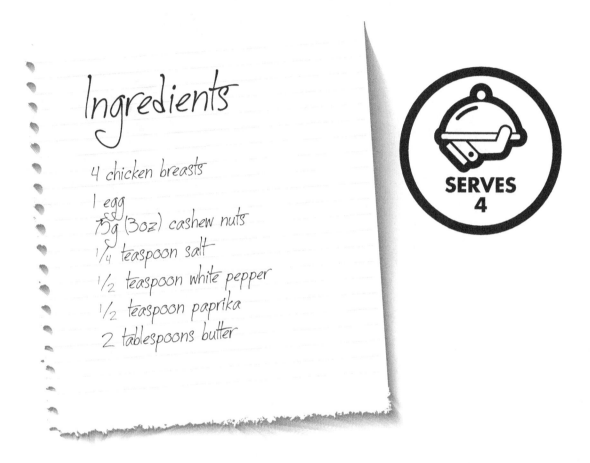

Ingredients

4 chicken breasts
1 egg
75g (3oz) cashew nuts
1/4 teaspoon salt
1/2 teaspoon white pepper
1/2 teaspoon paprika
2 tablespoons butter

SERVES 4

Method

Place the cashew nuts into a blender and process until they become fine. Transfer them to a plate, add the paprika, salt and pepper and mix well. In a separate bowl, beat the egg. Dip each of the chicken breasts into the egg, then into the cashew nut mixture and coat thoroughly. Heat the butter in a frying pan then add the chicken. Cook for about 5 minutes on each side until the chicken is golden and cooked thoroughly.

Almond & Lemon Baked Cod

SERVES 4

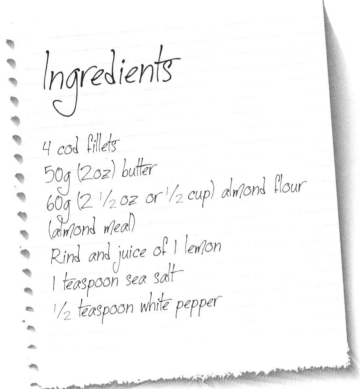

Ingredients

4 cod fillets
50g (2oz) butter
60g (2 ½ oz or ½ cup) almond flour (almond meal)
Rind and juice of 1 lemon
1 teaspoon sea salt
½ teaspoon white pepper

Method

Melt the butter in a saucepan and add the lemon juice and rind then set aside. On a plate, combine together the almond flour, salt and pepper. Dip the cod fillets into the lemon butter mixture then dunk in the almond flour making sure they are well coated. Lay out the fish on a baking tray. Bake in the oven at 180C/350F for around 25 minutes, or until the fish is flaky. Serve with a wedge of lemon.

Salmon, Herb Butter & Quinoa

SERVES 4

Ingredients

200g (7oz) quinoa
75g (3oz) butter
2 tablespoons fresh dill, chopped
1 tablespoon fresh chives, chopped
1 lemon, rind and juice
4 salmon steaks
1 tablespoon olive oil
Sea salt
Freshly ground black pepper

Method

Boil the quinoa for around 15 minutes until soft but firm then drain it. Combine the butter, chives, dill, lemon and lemon rind. Season with salt and pepper. Heat the olive oil in a pan. Add the salmon steaks and cook for 3-4 minutes on each side. Squeeze the lemon juice into the quinoa and season with salt and pepper. Serve the salmon onto plates and top with the lemon and herb butter. Place a helping of quinoa on the side.

Beef Stroganoff

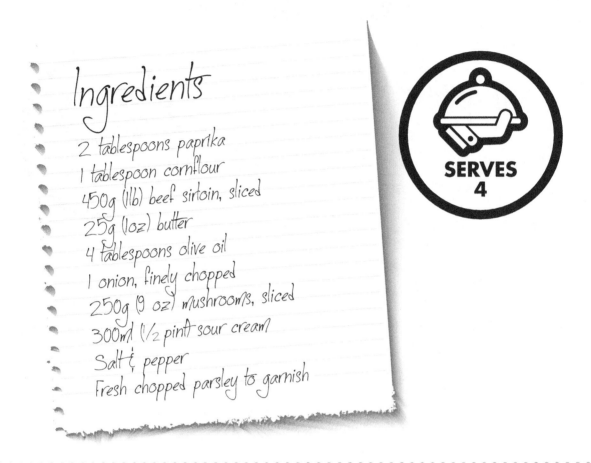

Ingredients

2 tablespoons paprika
1 tablespoon cornflour
450g (1lb) beef sirloin, sliced
25g (1oz) butter
4 tablespoons olive oil
1 onion, finely chopped
250g (9 oz) mushrooms, sliced
300ml (½ pint) sour cream
Salt & pepper
Fresh chopped parsley to garnish

SERVES 4

Method

Melt the butter and 2 tablespoons of the olive oil in a pan. Add the onion and cook for 5 minutes until soft. Add the mushrooms and cook for another 5 minutes. Remove the onions and mushrooms to a bowl and leave the oil in the pan. In a bowl, combine the paprika and cornflour then coat the beef in it. Add the remaining 2 tablespoons of olive oil and add the beef. Fry until browned. Reduce the heat and return the mushrooms and onions to the pan. Add the sour cream and heat gently it. Season with salt and pepper. Serve with rice and a sprinkling of parsley.

Chicken & Sweet Potato Pie

Ingredients

- 2 sweet potatoes, peeled and sliced
- 450g (1lb) chicken, diced
- 1 onion, chopped finely
- 2 carrots, chopped
- 1 teaspoon dried thyme
- 400ml (14fl oz) gluten-free chicken stock (broth)
- 150g (5oz) broccoli
- 1 garlic clove, crushed
- 1 teaspoon cornflour
- 2 teaspoons olive oil
- 1 tablespoon butter
- Sea salt and pepper

SERVES 4

Method

Heat the olive oil in a pan and fry the chicken for 5 minutes. Transfer to a bowl. Add the broccoli, onion and carrots and fry until they soften. Add the thyme and garlic. Cook for 1 minute. Sprinkle in the cornflour, stir well then add the chicken stock. Add the chicken to the pan then reduce the heat and simmer for 10 minutes. Transfer it all to an ovenproof casserole dish. Boil the sweet potatoes for 10-15 minutes, drain and mash them with butter and season with salt and pepper. Spread it over the chicken and vegetables. Bake in the oven at 200C/400F for 35-40 minutes. Remove, serve and enjoy.

Gluten-Free Nut Loaf

Ingredients

125g (4oz or 1 cup) walnuts
125g (4oz or 1 cup) hazelnuts
1 carrot, finely chopped
2 sticks celery, finely chopped
1 onion, finely chopped
125g (4oz or 1 cup) red lentils
125g (4oz or 1 1/2 cups) mushrooms, finely chopped
1 egg, beaten
50g (2oz or 1/4 cup) butter
2 teaspoons mild curry powder
2 teaspoons tomato puree (paste)
4 tablespoons fresh parsley, chopped
150ml (5fl oz) water
1 teaspoon sea salt

SERVES 4-6

Method

Steep the lentils in cold water for 1 hour. Heat the butter in a pan and add the carrot, celery, onion, mushrooms and curry powder. Fry for 5 minutes. Blitz the nuts in a food processor, and set aside. Drain and rinse the lentils, place them in a bowl and add the nuts. Stir in the vegetables, tomato puree (paste), egg, parsley, water and salt. Grease and line a large loaf tin with parchment paper. Put the mixture into a loaf tin and smooth out. Cover with foil. Bake in the oven at 190C/375F for 60-90 minutes. Let it stand for 10 minutes and turn onto a serving plate.

Chicken & Red Pepper Risotto

Ingredients

300g (11oz) risotto rice (Arborio)
1200ml (2 pints) warm gluten-free chicken stock (broth)
125g (4oz) cooked chicken, chopped
1 onion, chopped
1 red pepper (bell pepper), chopped
125g (4oz) spinach
1 tablespoon olive oil
Salt & black pepper

SERVES 4

Method

Heat the olive oil and a saucepan. Add the onion and red pepper (bell pepper). Cook for around 5 minutes until they have softened. Add the rice to the pan, stir and cook for 2 minutes, until the rice is coated in oil. Slowly add the stock (broth) while stirring and adding a little at a time until all the liquid has been absorbed, around 20 minutes. Add to the pan the spinach and chicken. Cook until the spinach has wilted - around 2 minutes. Season and serve.

Feta & Butterbean Cakes

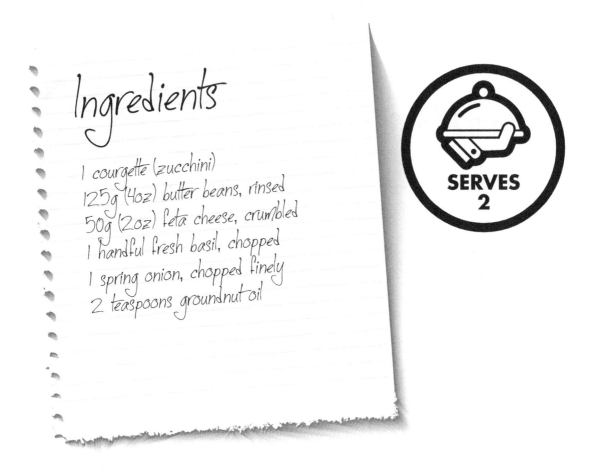

Ingredients

1 courgette (zucchini)
125g (4oz) butter beans, rinsed
50g (2oz) feta cheese, crumbled
1 handful fresh basil, chopped
1 spring onion, chopped finely
2 teaspoons groundnut oil

SERVES
2

Method

Grate the courgette (zucchini), then using a tea towel, or your hand, squeeze all the liquid from it. Leave to drain in a colander. Removing the excess liquid from the courgette will prevent the cakes from being bitter. In a large bowl, mash the butter beans, basil, spring onion, courgette (zucchini) and feta cheese. Combine them together well. Divide the mixture and using your hand, mould it into little patties. Place in the fridge for 10 minutes to firm up. Coat a frying pan with the oil and cook the patties on either side for around a minute. Remove them to a baking sheet and bake in the oven for 10 minutes at 220C/425F.

Melting Middle
Cheese Burgers

Ingredients

40g (1 (1/2 oz) chunk of Cheddar cheese
250g (9 oz) lean minced beef
(ground beef)
2 tablespoons fresh parsley,
finely chopped
Freshly ground black pepper
1 tablespoon groundnut oil

SERVES 2

Method

In a bowl, break-up the cheese and roll into 4 balls. In a separate bowl, mix the beef, parsley and black pepper then divide the mixture into 4. Roll into small balls. Make a deep well in the middle of each ball and place the cheese ball inside. Cover with meat and seal it so that no cheese is visible inside and flatten them slightly. Repeat for the burgers. Heat the oil in a frying pan over a high heat. Add the burgers and quickly brown for about 1 minute on each side. Reduce the heat and cook for around 3 minutes on each side.

Ginger Chicken

Ingredients

4 chicken breasts
2 tablespoons honey
225g (8oz) mushrooms, sliced
1 bunch of spring onions (scallions) finely chopped
3 cloves of garlic, crushed
2 (½ cm (1 inch) chunk of ginger root, finely chopped
½ teaspoon ground cinnamon
1 tablespoon olive oil
Rind and juice of 1 orange
1 orange cut into wedges for garnish

SERVES 4

Method

Preheat the oven to 190C/375F. Heat the oil in a frying pan. Add the chicken and cook for 2-3 minutes. Transfer the chicken to a casserole dish. In a bowl, mix together the honey, garlic, cinnamon, ginger, orange juice and rind. Pour the mixture onto the chicken. Place it in the oven for 10 minutes. Remove from the oven and add the mushrooms, spring onions and return to the oven for 15-20 minutes. Serve with rice and a wedge of orange to garnish.

DESSERTS, SWEET TREATS & SNACKS

Gluten-Free Scones

Ingredients

200g (7oz) gluten-free plain flour (all-purpose flour)
2 tablespoons caster sugar
2 teaspoons baking powder
25g (1oz) butter, chilled
120ml (4fl oz) double cream
120ml (4fl oz) water
milk, to brush
Pinch of salt

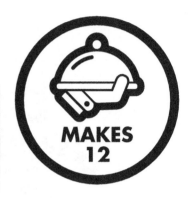

MAKES
12

Method

Combine together the flour, sugar, baking powder and a pinch of salt in a bowl. Cut flakes of butter and rub into the flour mixture with your fingers. Make a well in the centre of the mixture. Add the cream and water. Use a flat bladed knife to mix it together. Transfer to a flat surface and gently knead until the mixture just comes together, being careful to not over knead. Gently flatten the mixture to around 2cm (1 inch) thick. Use a round cutter to cut 12 rounds from the dough. Preheat oven to 200C/400F. Place the scones on a lightly greased baking sheet. Brush lightly with milk. Bake at 200C/400F for 20 minutes or until golden and serve.

Banana Bread

Ingredients

300g (11oz) rice flour
100g (3½ oz) butter
4 bananas
200ml (7fl oz) milk (soya, rice
or coconut milk works too)
4 teaspoons baking powder (gluten-free)
2 eggs

SERVES 4-6

Method

Place all the ingredients into a food processor and process until smooth. Line a large loaf tin with greaseproof parchment paper. Spread the mixture into the tin. Heat the oven to 180C/350F. Bake for 35 minutes. Check to see if it's done using a skewer which should come out clean. Turn out of the tin and allow it to cool before serving.

Chocolate Florentines

Ingredients

2 tablespoons blanched almonds

150g (5oz) chocolate, minimum 75% cocoa

2 tablespoons shelled unsalted pistachio nuts

2 tablespoons dried cranberries

1 tablespoon toasted coconut flakes

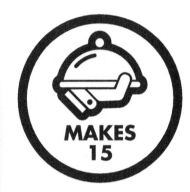

MAKES 15

Method

Line several baking sheets with grease-proof paper. Place the chocolate in a heatproof bowl over a saucepan of gently simmering water and heat it until melted. Pour spoonfuls of chocolate onto a baking sheet to make a round disc shape. Do this for all the melted chocolate. Before it sets, place equal amounts of the dried fruit, nuts and coconut flakes onto each disc. Leave to set for 2-3 hours.

Panna Cotta & Raspberries

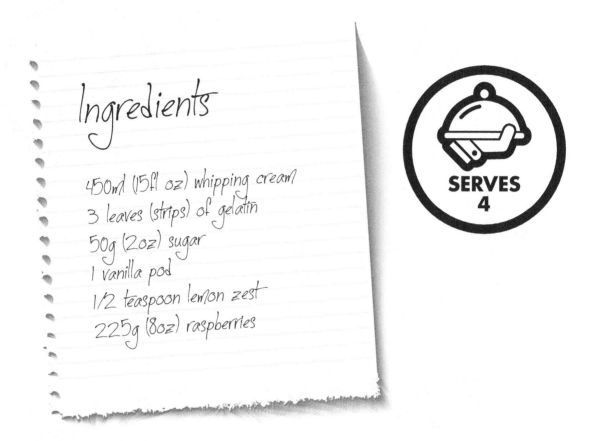

Ingredients

450ml (15fl oz) whipping cream
3 leaves (strips) of gelatin
50g (2oz) sugar
1 vanilla pod
1/2 teaspoon lemon zest
225g (8oz) raspberries

SERVES 4

Method

Put the cream and sugar in a saucepan. Cut the vanilla pod in half, scrape out the seeds and add to the saucepan. Heat the cream for about 3 minutes. Soften the gelatin in a bowl of cold water. Remove the saucepan from the heat. Add the gelatin and stir until it dissolves. Add the lemon zest and mix. Pour out the vanilla cream mixture into 4 moulds or ramekin dishes. Chill for 4-5 hours. When you are ready to serve, dip the moulds briefly in hot water and turn out onto a plate. Serve with raspberries.

Strawberry Cream Lollies

Ingredients

360ml (12 fl oz)
plain yogurt (unflavoured)
150g (5oz) strawberries

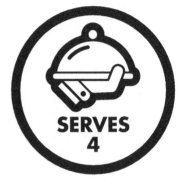

SERVES
4

Method

Set aside a few of the strawberries to add whole to the lollies. Blitz the remaining strawberries in a food processor until smooth. Add the yogurt to the strawberries, stirring slowly to achieve a swirly effect. Add in the remaining whole berries and stir. Spoon the mix into ice-lolly moulds. Add a few berries as you fill the moulds. Transfer the moulds to the freezer for at least 2 hours until they are frozen solid.

Figs, Honey & Yogurt

Ingredients

4 tablespoons plain
(unflavoured) yogurt
2 tablespoons honey
8 figs

SERVES
4

Method

Cut the figs in half and place in a hot frying pan with the skin facing down. Cook them for 10 minutes until the skin darkens. Place the figs onto plates. Top with a spoonful of yogurt and drizzle with honey.

Summer Pudding

Ingredients

500g (1lb 2oz) mixed berries, blueberries, strawberries, redcurrants, raspberries, blackcurrants

60g (2½ oz) caster sugar (or super-fine sugar)

18 slices gluten-free bread

Yogurt or crème fraiche to serve

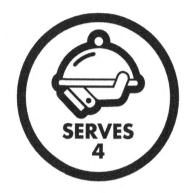

SERVES 4

Method

Put half of the berries into a bowl and sprinkle with half of the sugar. Place the remaining berries in a food processor with the remaining sugar and blitz until smooth. Strain through a sieve. Line 4 x 200ml (7fl oz) dariole moulds with cling film (plastic wrap). Using a pastry cutter, cut out 4 circles of bread to line the base of each mould. Remove crusts from the rest of the bread and cut into 3cm strips. Dip the bread circles into the fruit puree and put in the base of the mould. Dip the remaining bread in the fruit puree and line the sides of the mould. Fill the moulds with whole berries. Finally, dip the large rounds in fruit puree and place on top of the moulds. Cover with cling film (plastic wrap), place a plate or chopping board over the bottom and chill. Serve with leftover puree and yogurt or crème fraiche.

Lemon & Polenta Cake

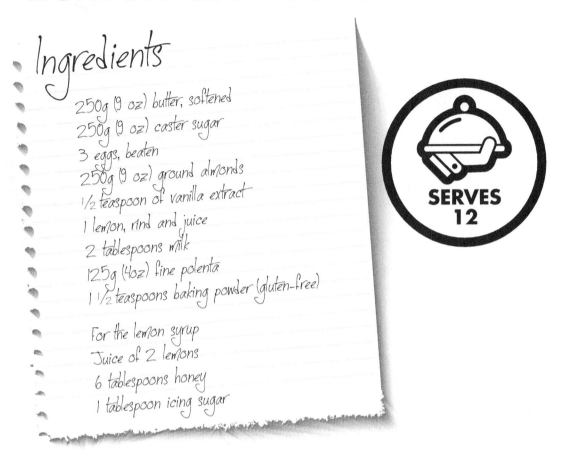

Ingredients

250g (9 oz) butter, softened
250g (9 oz) caster sugar
3 eggs, beaten
250g (9 oz) ground almonds
1/2 teaspoon of vanilla extract
1 lemon, rind and juice
2 tablespoons milk
125g (4oz) fine polenta
1 1/2 teaspoons baking powder (gluten-free)

For the lemon syrup
Juice of 2 lemons
6 tablespoons honey
1 tablespoon icing sugar

SERVES 12

Method

Beat the butter and sugar until light and creamy. Slowly add the beaten eggs and combine. Fold in the ground almonds, vanilla, lemon juice and rind, milk, polenta and baking powder. Grease and line a 23cm (9 in) cake tin. Pour the mixture into the tin and smooth it. Place in the oven and bake at 160C/325F for 50 mins-1hr. Test it with a skewer which should come out clean. Remove from the oven and leave it in the tin.

For the syrup, put the lemon juice and honey in a saucepan and stir in the icing sugar until it has dissolved. Spoon the syrup over the cake while the cake and the syrup are hot.

Chocolate & Orange Mousse

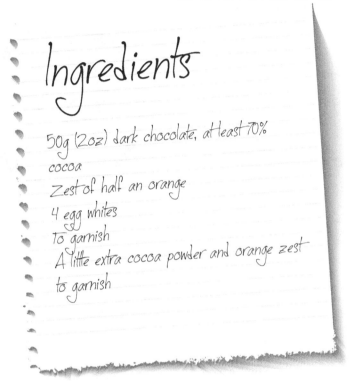

Ingredients

50g (2oz) dark chocolate, at least 70% cocoa

Zest of half an orange

4 egg whites

To garnish

A little extra cocoa powder and orange zest to garnish

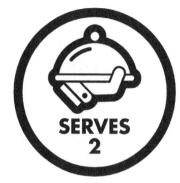

SERVES 2

Method

Melt the chocolate in a heatproof bowl, placed over a saucepan of gently simmering water. Keep the base of the bowl out of the water. Once melted, leave to cool slightly. Add the orange zest to the melted chocolate and mix together. Whisk the egg whites in a bowl until they form soft peaks. Fold them into the melted chocolate. Spoon the mixture into two small cups or ramekin dishes. Scatter a little orange zest onto the mousse and dust with cocoa powder. Chill before serving.

Coconut & Chocolate Truffles

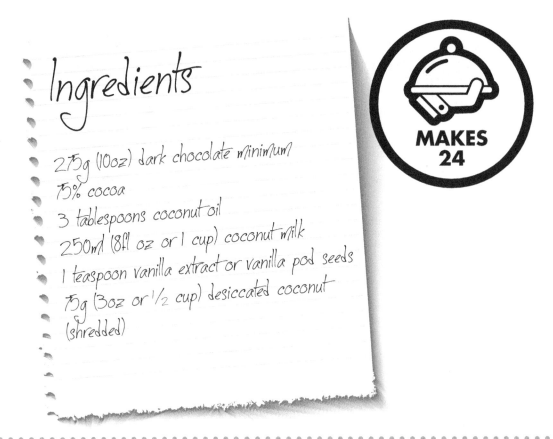

MAKES
24

Ingredients

275g (10oz) dark chocolate minimum
75% cocoa
3 tablespoons coconut oil
250ml (8fl oz or 1 cup) coconut milk
1 teaspoon vanilla extract or vanilla pod seeds
75g (3oz or 1/2 cup) desiccated coconut
(shredded)

Method

Break the chocolate into pieces and place in a medium sized bowl with the coconut oil. In a saucepan, heat the coconut milk until it is simmering. Pour the coconut milk over the chocolate and coconut oil. Add the vanilla and combine the ingredients by gently stirring. Once it's ready, scoop out balls of chocolate using a melon-baller. If necessary, roll it in your palms to smooth the chocolate ball. Put the coconut in a small plastic bag and roll the truffle to coat it. Alternatively, coat the truffles in cocoa powder using the same technique. Place the truffles in small paper cases, ready to eat.

Chocolate Almond Cake

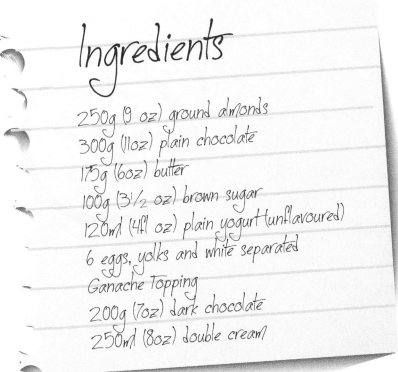

Ingredients

250g (9 oz) ground almonds
300g (11oz) plain chocolate
175g (6oz) butter
100g (3½ oz) brown sugar
120ml (4fl oz) plain yogurt (unflavoured)
6 eggs, yolks and white separated
Ganache Topping
200g (7oz) dark chocolate
250ml (8oz) double cream

SERVES 6-8

Method

Grease and line a 25cm (10 inch) cake tin with greaseproof (parchment) paper. Put a mixing bowl over a saucepan of gently simmering water. Add the 300g of chocolate to the bowl and stir until melted. Add the 175g (6oz) butter and combine with the chocolate. Remove from the heat and set aside. Whisk the egg whites until they are stiff and set aside.

Place the brown sugar and egg yolks in a bowl and whisk them together. Stir in the chocolate and butter. Add in the yogurt and almonds. Stir well, then fold in the whisked egg whites. Pour into the cake tin. Bake in the middle of the oven at 180C/350F for 60-70 minutes. Test with a skewer before removing. Let the cake cool in the tin then remove it.

Topping – Break the chocolate into a bowl. Heat the cream in a saucepan. When nearly boiling, pour the cream onto the chocolate and mix until smooth. Cover the cake with the topping and enjoy.

Date Muffins

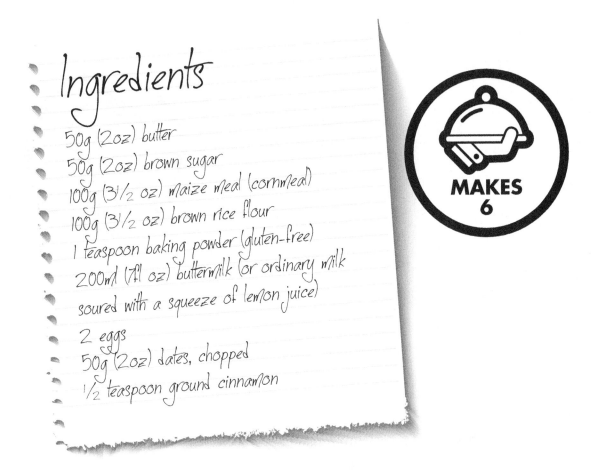

Ingredients

50g (2oz) butter
50g (2oz) brown sugar
100g (3½ oz) maize meal (cornmeal)
100g (3½ oz) brown rice flour
1 teaspoon baking powder (gluten-free)
200ml (7fl oz) buttermilk (or ordinary milk
soured with a squeeze of lemon juice)

2 eggs
50g (2oz) dates, chopped
½ teaspoon ground cinnamon

MAKES 6

Method

Preheat the oven to 200C/400F. Lightly grease a 6 hole muffin tin. Mix the butter and sugar together until creamy. Add the eggs one at a time and combine with the butter and sugar until smooth. Add the buttermilk and stir. In a separate bowl, place the rice flour, maize meal, cinnamon and baking powder and mix together. Slowly fold the dry ingredients into the butter, eggs and milk then add the chopped dates. Spoon the mixture into the muffin tin. Bake in the oven for 25-30 minutes, or until thoroughly cooked. Place on a wire rack and serve when still slightly warm.

Rice Pudding With Cinnamon & Nuts

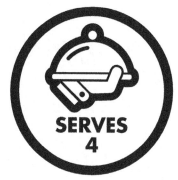

SERVES 4

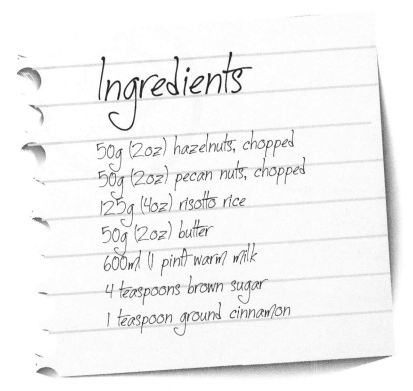

Ingredients

50g (2oz) hazelnuts, chopped
50g (2oz) pecan nuts, chopped
125g (4oz) risotto rice
50g (2oz) butter
600ml (1 pint) warm milk
4 teaspoons brown sugar
1 teaspoon ground cinnamon

Method

Heat a saucepan and add the nuts. Toast the nuts until golden then set aside. Heat the butter in a saucepan and add the rice. Stir and cook for around 1 minute. Slowly add the warm milk to the rice, stirring continuously. Add the sugar and cinnamon and simmer gently for around 20 minutes. Serve the rice pudding into bowls and sprinkle with the toasted nuts.

Sugar-Free Chocolate & Nut Brittle

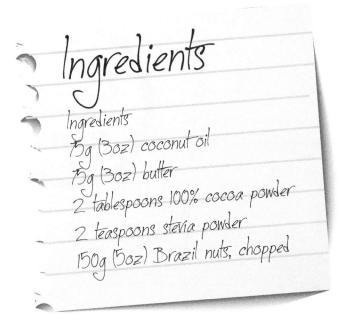

Ingredients

Ingredients
75g (3oz) coconut oil
75g (3oz) butter
2 tablespoons 100% cocoa powder
2 teaspoons stevia powder
150g (5oz) Brazil nuts, chopped

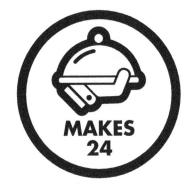

MAKES
24

Method

Melt the butter and coconut oil in a saucepan. Stir in the cocoa powder and stevia and mix until smooth. Place half of the chopped Brazil nuts in the bottom of a small dish or small loaf tin. Pour on half the chocolate mixture. Sprinkle on the remaining chopped nuts and add the remaining chocolate. Chill for at least an hour until the chocolate is hard. Using a knife, cut it into 24 small pieces, or break it into large rough chunks and serve. The coconut oil in the chocolate will melt in a warm room, so it needs to be kept chilled until ready to eat.

Note: You can use shop bought chocolate instead if you don't wish to make your recipe sugar-free. Simply heat the chocolate in a bowl over a saucepan of gently simmering water then pour half onto the Brazils and proceed as per the instructions.

Beetroot Chips

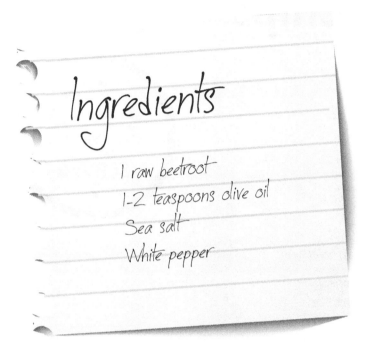

Ingredients

1 raw beetroot
1-2 teaspoons olive oil
Sea salt
White pepper

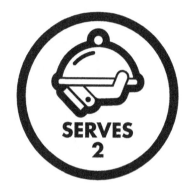

SERVES 2

Method

Peel the beetroot and cut into thin slices of no more than 2mm thick. Coat the beetroot with olive oil and season with salt and pepper. Lay them out in a single layer onto a lightly greased baking tray. Transfer to the oven and bake at 200C/400F for 10 minutes or until they are crisp and golden. Let them sit on kitchen paper to drain off excess oil. Serve with dips.

Courgette (Zucchini) Chips

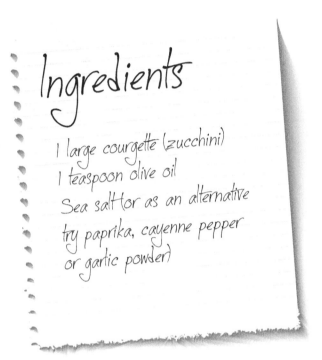

Ingredients

1 large courgette (zucchini)
1 teaspoon olive oil
Sea salt(or as an alternative
try paprika, cayenne pepper
or garlic powder)

SERVES
2

Method

Slice the courgette (zucchini) into thin circles, around the thickness of a coin. Place them in a bowl, add a teaspoon of olive oil and seasoning. Toss to lightly coat them. Line a baking sheet with foil, and lay out the slices onto the sheet. Preheat the oven to 220C/425F and bake the chips for 30 minutes, turning once. Remove when crispy and golden. Serve and eat immediately.

Curry Flavour Nuts

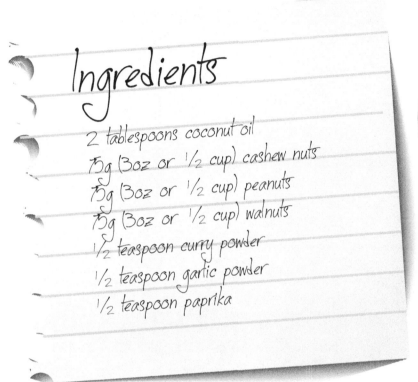

Ingredients

2 tablespoons coconut oil

75g (3oz or ½ cup) cashew nuts

75g (3oz or ½ cup) peanuts

75g (3oz or ½ cup) walnuts

½ teaspoon curry powder

½ teaspoon garlic powder

½ teaspoon paprika

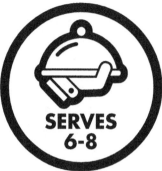

SERVES 6-8

Method

Heat the coconut oil in a large frying pan. Add all of the nuts, the curry powder, garlic and paprika to the hot pan. Stir and cook for around 7-8 minutes. Store or serve as a party nibble or snack. Try substituting the spices for cinnamon for a sweeter variation.

SAUCES AND CONDIMENTS

Aioli (Garlic Mayonnaise)

Ingredients

1 large egg yolk
4 cloves of garlic, crushed
1 tablespoon lemon juice
175ml (6fl oz) olive oil

1 tablespoon fresh chives, finely chopped
Salt and white pepper

Method

Whisk the egg yolk in a bowl. Add the garlic, lemon juice and season with salt and pepper. Gradually add the olive oil, a little at a time, until it's all combined and you have a smooth thick sauce. Add the chives and stir. Serve with fish or meat dishes.

Tomato Salsa

Ingredients

2 ripe tomatoes, finely chopped
½ red onion, finely chopped
1 stick of celery, finely chopped
1 tablespoon fresh coriander (cilant-

ro), finely chopped
1 clove of garlic, crushed
1 tablespoon olive oil
2 tablespoons lemon juice

Method

Place all the ingredients into a bowl and mix together. Chill before serving. As a variation you can try adding a tablespoon of basil instead of coriander. It makes a great accompaniment to chicken dishes and salads.

Spicy Pineapple Salsa

Ingredients

1 fresh ripe pineapple, diced finely
½ red onion, finely chopped
2.5cm (1inch) chunk of fresh ginger,
peel and finely chopped

½ teaspoon garam masala
½ teaspoon ground cumin
1 tablespoon coriander leaves or mint,
finely chopped

Method

Place all the ingredients in a bowl and mix. Allow to sit and infuse for 20 minutes before serving.

Gluten-Free Ketchup

Ingredients

175ml (6fl oz) tomato paste
2 tablespoons of onion powder
1 teaspoon garlic powder
½ teaspoon ground sea salt
150ml (5fl oz) apple cider vinegar

60ml (2fl oz) water
⅛ teaspoon of ground cloves
⅛ teaspoon cinnamon
⅛ teaspoon allspice
⅛ teaspoon pepper

Method

Place all the ingredients in a bowl and stir until smooth. Keep the ketchup in a glass jar in the refrigerator, ready to use.

111

Mustard Vinaigrette

Ingredients

4 tablespoons olive oil
1 tablespoon apple cider vinegar (or lemon juice)
1 teaspoon mustard
1 clove of garlic, crushed
1/4 teaspoon sea salt
Freshly ground black pepper

Method

Mix the ingredients together in a bowl or shaker before serving and use with fresh salads.

Walnut Vinaigrette

Ingredients

4 tablespoons walnut oil
2-3 tablespoons apple cider vinegar
Sea salt
Freshly ground black pepper

Method

Stir the oil and vinegar together and season with sea salt. Can be stored in the fridge or used immediately.

Vegetable Stock

Ingredients

1 large onion, peel and chopped
2 carrots, peeled and chopped
1 stalk celery, chopped
1 leek, washed and chopped
2 cloves garlic, chopped
1 tablespoon parsley
1 tablespoon thyme
1 tablespoon tarragon
1 bay leaf
1 teaspoon sea salt
1 teaspoon white pepper
2 litres (3 pints) water

Method

Add all the ingredients to a large soup saucepan and cover with the water and bring to the bowl. Reduce the heat and simmer for 45 minutes. Allow to cool. Strain the vegetable stock and place in containers, ready to be placed in the freezer.

Chicken Stock (Broth)

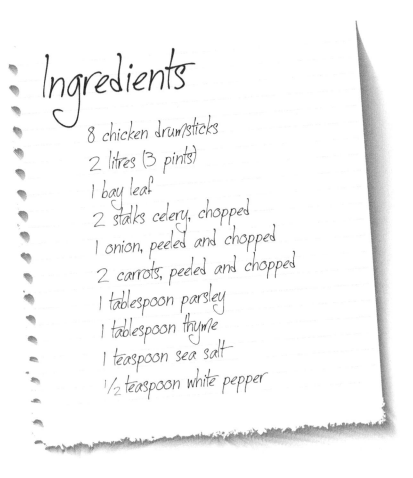

Ingredients

8 chicken drumsticks
2 litres (3 pints)
1 bay leaf
2 stalks celery, chopped
1 onion, peeled and chopped
2 carrots, peeled and chopped
1 tablespoon parsley
1 tablespoon thyme
1 teaspoon sea salt
1/2 teaspoon white pepper

Method

Place all the ingredients into a large soup saucepan, cover with the water and bring to the boil. Reduce to a low heat. Skim off any foam from the top of the pot. Simmer for 90 minutes. Allow to cool then strain the stock through a sieve and place in containers ready to be frozen. Use a draining spoon and remove the chicken. It can be saved and make into a curry or kept as a leftover meal to be added to stir fries or omelettes.

Onion Gravy

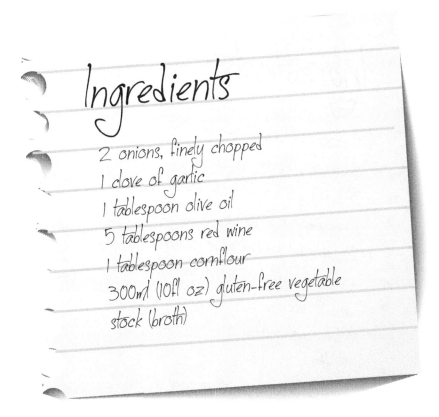

Ingredients

2 onions, finely chopped
1 clove of garlic
1 tablespoon olive oil
5 tablespoons red wine
1 tablespoon cornflour
300ml (10fl oz) gluten-free vegetable stock (broth)

Method

Heat the olive oil in a frying pan. Add the onions and garlic. Cook for 15 minutes until the onion is very soft. Stir in the red wine and reduce it down to half the amount of liquid. Sprinkle in the cornflour. Stir it really well while slowly adding the stock. Gently simmer while the gravy thickens. You can add extra water if it seems too thick.

Tomato & Herb Sauce

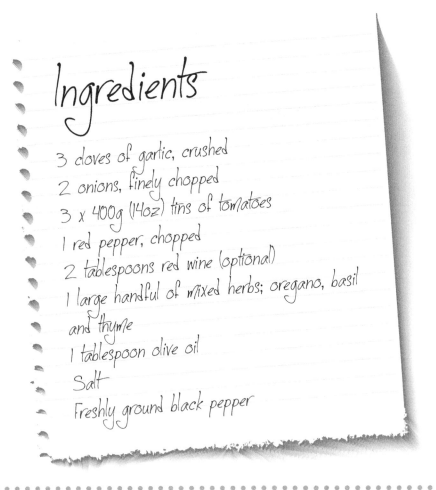

Ingredients

3 cloves of garlic, crushed
2 onions, finely chopped
3 x 400g (14oz) tins of tomatoes
1 red pepper, chopped
2 tablespoons red wine (optional)
1 large handful of mixed herbs; oregano, basil and thyme
1 tablespoon olive oil
Salt
Freshly ground black pepper

Method

Heat the olive oil in a pan. Add the garlic and onions. Cook until soft and translucent. Pour in the tomatoes and add the red pepper to the onions. Add the red wine and cook for 15 minutes. Add the mixed herbs and season with salt and pepper. This makes a large batch which can be frozen and used for pasta sauces and pizza toppings.

Made in the USA
Monee, IL
17 April 2023

31993034R00070